To Jacob +
Samuel

Best Wishes !

[signature]

My life as a sibling to chronic disease
a memoir by Randall Stark Beach

SHADOW
CHILD

outskirts
press

TABLE OF CONTENTS

PART TWO: SHADOW CHILD

PART THREE: OBSERVATIONS AND WORDS OF ADVICE

ACKNOWLEDGEMENTS

I wish to express my sincere gratitude to the following individuals who helped to make this book possible: my wife, Sarah, whose tireless encouragement and proofreading got me over the finish line; my mother, Lois, and my brother, Jon, both took time to read early manuscripts and provide precious insights; Bernard Shaw, who lent a steadying hand whenever the boat began to rock a bit much; and my editor, Julie Lang, who was invaluable to the finished product.

INTRODUCTION

Imagine you are seven years old. Your best friend is your four-year-old brother. Suddenly, you are told your brother is in the hospital because he has a disease that has a name you can't pronounce and that won't go away. In a youthful instant, your family and your life are turned upside down. Routines change, and your parents focus on the often-overwhelming needs of your sick brother. Within days, you find that the world is topsy-turvy and that you are in the shadows.

Perhaps you—like my brother, my parents, and me—do not need to imagine such a scenario. The story of two adults and their children suddenly confronted with a medical diagnosis that immediately changes all of their lives is all too common. The story is both sad and happy. It is, in short, real life.

While the pages that follow are full of tales about my brother, my parents, other family members, and friends who joined us on our unexpected journey, you will not find a villainous person. I cannot stress enough my conviction that no one in this story is a bad actor. Instead,

III

this is a tale of genuine people trying to do their best while coping with a life-changing, chronic disease inflicted on the youngest member of a modern nuclear family.

If there is a villain within these pages, it is the disease, diabetes mellitus. I try, as a rule, not to be overly generous with anthropomorphic properties, but diabetes has been a negative part of my life for more than thirty-six years. Diabetes severely altered my relationship with my parents and my brother. It erased a normal sibling relationship and replaced it with a quasi-parental mutation. When I think of the disease in this light, it is a bad actor. Diabetes is the villain.

If you are intimately familiar with this particular bad actor, feel free to skip ahead. For those less familiar with the disease, let me introduce you to my family's nemesis.

Diabetes mellitus is a term for a group of diseases that includes type 1 diabetes, type 2 diabetes, and gestational diabetes.[1] According to the American Diabetes Association, approximately 29.1 million people in the United States have some form of diabetes.[2] Of these, about 208,000 children and teenagers are inflicted with the disease.

Today's news is rife with stories of type 2 diabetes, the occurrence of which has begun to rise to epidemic proportions in many parts of the world. Type 2 diabetes is characterized by the body's resistance to a hormone that regulates the blood sugar levels within our bodies. People generally treat the disease through medication and dietary changes. Type 2 diabetes is prevalent in overweight people and used to be referred to in medical circles as adult-onset diabetes. Sadly, with

---

1   Gestational diabetes occurs during a woman's pregnancy and often disappears when the child is delivered.
2   "Statistics about Diabetes," American Diabetes Association, last modified September 10, 2014, accessed November 12, 2014, http://www.diabetes.org/diabetes-basics/statistics.

increased numbers for childhood obesity, this moniker is no longer appropriate.

Type 1 diabetes is the form that most often strikes young children and sometimes adults. The Juvenile Diabetes Research Foundation estimates that more than fifteen thousand children and fifteen thousand adults are diagnosed with type 1 diabetes in the United States each year.[3]

Type 1 diabetes is characterized by the pancreas's complete inability to produce insulin.[4] Insulin is the hormone charged with regulating the absorption of glucose (blood sugar) by muscle and fat cells. It is produced in specialized beta cells found within the pancreas and secreted into the bloodstream from that organ. Glucose is critical to the human body because it is used by the body's cells for energy, to make other necessary molecules, or for fuel storage. If your body cannot produce insulin, it cannot process glucose. If your body cannot properly process glucose, it fails.

In most cases, type 1 diabetes is an autoimmune condition. That is, the body's T cells attack and destroy the insulin-producing beta cells of the pancreas. At present, it is believed that type 1 diabetes requires both a genetic disposition and an environmental cause. The environmental trigger is often a viral infection of some sort. There is no known preventative measure against the disease, and there is no cure.

People with type 1 diabetes are forced to introduce insulin daily into their body, either through injections or via an insulin pump. Until the last decade or so, insulin was administered solely through daily insulin shots. The number of required daily insulin shots differs from

---

3   "Type 1 Diabetes Facts," Juvenile Diabetes Research Foundation, accessed November 12, 2014, http://jdrf.org/about-jdrf/fact-sheets/type-1-diabetes-facts.
4   Insulin was discovered in 1921 by two Canadians, Dr. Frederick Banting and his medical student, Charles Best.

individual to individual and is affected by a variety of other factors, including activity levels. In the best cases, insulin shots are taken in the morning and in the evening.

Failure to take insulin shots or administer the proper amount of insulin results in either hyperglycemia (high blood sugar) or hypoglycemia (low blood sugar). Of the two conditions, hyperglycemia presents the greatest danger. High blood sugar in a person with type 1 diabetes can result from eating too much or not taking enough insulin. Without treatment, hyperglycemia leads to ketoacidosis,[5] a condition also known as diabetic coma. When a diabetic's body does not have enough insulin to break down glucose into fuel, the body begins to break down its own fat stores for energy. This process results in the creation of ketones. The buildup of ketones in the blood leads to coma and, possibly, death.

Hypoglycemia is slightly less dangerous than hyperglycemia. Low blood sugar results from too much insulin and not enough glucose in the bloodstream. Hypoglycemia is also known as an "insulin reaction," and I use this term, or simply "reaction," throughout the pages that follow. Symptoms of such a reaction include shakiness, dizziness, hunger, pale skin color, sudden mood changes, crying, screaming, clumsiness, confusion, and sometimes seizures.

Loss of control and confusion can occur as a result of the low blood sugar condition. If untreated, a diabetic who is having an insulin reaction is likely to pass out. These effects can easily lead to dangers such as perilous falls and car crashes.

Eventually, the hypoglycemic body kicks in and releases hormones to bring the body back into balance. However, these hormones are subject to a degree of natural interference within the body. In extreme cases,

---

5   "DKA (Ketoacidosis) & Ketones," American Diabetes Association, last modified March 12, 2014, accessed November 12, 2014, http://www.diabetes.org/living-with-diabetes/complications/ketoacidosis-dka.html.

even though it may not be as life threatening as hyperglycemia, untreated hypoglycemia may result in coma and brain damage.

In addition to hyperglycemia and hypoglycemia, diabetes brings many complications into the lives of its victims. Some of these complications can be avoided through careful management of the disease, but others seem nearly inevitable given enough time. Common diabetic complications include eye problems and even eventual blindness, skin infections, loss of circulation in the feet and legs that often leads to amputations, heart disease, high blood pressure, increased instances of gum diseases, kidney disease, strokes, and hearing loss.

One hundred years ago, type 1 diabetes was considered a terminal illness. Even with the state-of-the-art treatment available today, diabetes takes a severe toll on those it inflicts. In 2010, diabetes directly caused or indirectly contributed to approximately 234,051 deaths in the United States, according to the American Diabetes Association.[6]

It is easy for outsiders to see the impact of a chronic disease such as type 1 diabetes on its youthful target—and on the parents who care for the child and help manage the disease. But the healthy sibling tends to be left out of the analysis.

Healthy siblings are often labeled as "lucky." We are seen solely as the children who were spared the devastating disease that their brother or sister has to deal with day in and day out. For some reason, it is assumed that we are untouched by the illness. We are, after all, the lucky ones.

In reality, healthy siblings suffer alongside our less healthy brothers and sisters. Our roles within the family structure are changed overnight. We take on more responsibility for our sick sibling, and for family

---

6   "Statistics about Diabetes," American Diabetes Association.

matters as a whole, than would normally be cast upon a child. We struggle to understand why our parents' attention is suddenly devoted to our brother or sister when it used to be shared so evenly. We spend time feeling guilty and wondering why the disease targeted our sibling and overlooked us. We fight back our jealousy and resentment as best we can, but it still comes out. We deal with tremendous fear. We are afraid for our sick sibling, and our sick sibling scares us.

All of these feelings are thrust upon us, yet most of us are left alone. We are forced to try and comprehend and cope with our new roles by ourselves. We are loved, but we are alone. We are shadow children.

PART ONE
DEMANDS OF DISEASE

Chapter One

---~~~---

MAKING TOAST

Sounds of terror pop my eyes open, jolting me from sleep. Glancing to my right, my fuzzy head registers the neon red numerals glowing from my alarm clock. 2:10 a.m. It's that time, I realize, and I wait for the second horrible wail to confirm my suspicion. It arrives in seconds: a sustained cry of naked terror. Almost simultaneously I hear the ruffle of bedding as my parents jump from underneath their covers and sprint down the hall. Despite familiarity, my heart begins to race and my throat tightens.

I am twelve years old. I am in my own bed, on the second floor of the house I have lived in all of my life. My entire immediate family is here: my parents and Jon, my nine-year-old brother. I am warm, the covers pulled up around me. I am also scared.

The screams of terror come from my brother. They continue at an increasing rate but decreasing volume. Between the screams and the occasional sobs, I hear the voices of my parents.

"It's okay Pudge," my dad repeatedly says in a voice mixed with sleep and panic, my brother's family nickname slipping from his lips.

"Jon. Jon, open up, come on," my mom says in a firm, determined voice, the same one she uses when telling me to sit down and do my homework.

I stay in my bed, sheltered by the covers for a minute or so more, and then decide it's time to get up and help. Pushing aside the blankets, I swing my legs down to the floor. The fog of early morning sleep has been swept away by the terrible noises coming from my brother's room. Adrenaline rules the hour now.

In my fuzzy dark blue pajamas with their nondescript football helmet pattern, I quickly walk out of my room into the hall, past my parents' now vacant bedroom, and turning, above the stairway to approach the doorway of Jon's room. I know what I will find inside. I have seen this scene so many times, but still I hesitate, fighting familiar fear.

Crossing the threshold, I stop at the expected scene. My brother sits on the edge of the bed, cowering in his red *Star Wars* pajamas. To the left of Jon sits my dad, his plain navy blue pajamas wrinkled from sleep. He perches on the edge of the bed with his arm around my brother, supporting him. Mom's white nightgown brushes Jon's knees as she half kneels, half stands in front of him. My parents' faces are intent and grave. My brother's mouth still releases those soul-wrenching screams.

Jon also shakes uncontrollably. My parents speak to each other in soft tones, with only hints of panic. My mom fights with my brother to keep his mouth open so that she can squeeze small packets of honey inside. If necessary, she squeezes the honey onto her fingers and shoves them into Jon's mouth, rubbing the sticky, sugary substance into the inside of his cheeks. She has been bitten before, but she continues without hesitation.

4

There is no need for me to stay still and soak in the all-too-familiar actions.

"I'll get the toast," I declare to the room in a voice still filled with sleep and now tinged with bit of fear.

"Okay, go ahead." The response is from my dad, his arms still supporting my brother's back.

Turning out of the doorway, I am glad to have something to do and even happier that the task requires me to leave Jon's bedroom. I hit the stairs and sleepily stumble my way to the first floor, heading for the dark kitchen.

Before I am out of earshot, I hear my mom's firm and unwavering voice once more. "Jon, look at me. Open your eyes, Jon, and look at me."

Flipping the light switch to the left of the doorway from the hall, I turn on the kitchen lights overhead. They're shockingly bright at that hour and remind me that I should be in bed, sleeping for another four hours or so. Instead, I am squinting and moving to the bread drawer. I am here making toast.

A rustle of fur, blanket, and metal tells me that I am not alone in the kitchen, even at this hour. Cassie, the dog gifted to my brother when he learned to give his own insulin shots, is in her crate in the adjacent laundry room. She stirs but does not get up. Even she is becoming used to this early morning routine.

From the bread drawer I pull out the loaf of white bread, open the plastic sleeve, and slide out the first two slices. Placing them in the nearby toaster, I remember to slide the button all the way down. I don't want to forget that again and try my parents' impatience. I take a deep breath, lean against the cold kitchen counter, and wait.

The silence of the kitchen is comforting. I am glad to be downstairs, away from my trembling, terrified brother. I don't want to be my parents, forcing honey down Jon's throat. I don't want to hear the sobs or screams from him. Making toast is my job, and I do it happily.

The toaster's "pop" reminds me that my job is only partly complete. Turning toward the toaster and the countertop, I remove a creamy white plate from the cupboard and gingerly take the hot slices of bread from the mouth of the toaster, placing them on the plate. I open the refrigerator for the butter and jelly. With a knife, I spread the butter first and then layers of jelly. I am generous with the jelly; I don't want to do this again before dawn.

With the toast buttered and jellied, I take the plate and march through the kitchen and hallway and back up the stairs. I hear Jon talking now. He is responding to Mom's questions. His confusion is gone. He knows where he is, who she is, who my dad is. He will be okay.

Toast in hand, I arrive again at the doorway to my brother's room. My dad is picking up the emptied honey packages from the floor. Mom is wiping Jon's sticky mouth with a wet washcloth. His eyes turn to me when I walk into the room. He is quiet now and his body is still. He is back in control, and back to being the brother I know so well.

My mom puts the washcloth down and takes the plate of toast from me. She thanks me but then reminds me that I can go back to bed. I stay for a few more minutes. Jon is talking again, answering more of Mom's reassuring questions.

Dad rises from the bed, places his hand on my shoulder as he passes me, and walks out of the room and into the adjacent bathroom. This too is part of our well-rehearsed, early morning routine. Having risen from bed so quickly in response to my brother's terror, my dad is sick to his stomach. It happens every time.

The first half of the toast is gone, and Jon busily shoves the second half into his mouth. He is smiling and looks content with the early morning snack. I say a weary goodnight to the room and leave my mom and brother sitting on the bed.

Returning to my bedroom, I slide back under the sheet and pull the blankets up around me. Before closing my eyes, I glance at the neon red numerals of my alarm clock. 2:53 a.m. It's funny how it always seems to take longer than it actually does.

Dad will be calling my name in just a few hours to get me up for school. Closing my eyes, I hope for quick sleep.

Chapter Two

Chapter Two

~

FAMILY

My father, Charles Randall Beach, was born on August 4, 1947, in the middle of the hustle and bustle of postwar New York City. His stint as a city boy was brief, because my grandparents moved from New York shortly after my father was born, trying Poultney, Vermont, and Round Lake, New York, before settling in Lancaster, Pennsylvania. Those few months in 1947 were the first and last time that my father lived in the big city.

While there are many interesting tales surrounding my father's family, only a brief sketch is necessary for you to better understand his role in my story. The Beaches came to America in the 1640s, though our ancestry includes William Bradford, the first governor of Plymouth Colony, as well as several successful businessmen.

By my grandparents' generation, the family fortunes had cycled up and down, and careers for both parents were more common, particularly through the war years. After writing for the Associated Press, my grandmother, Rosemary, spent the rest of her working life as a librarian. My grandfather, Tom, worked in the insurance and mortgage industries, following in his stepfather's footsteps, and always had a hand in real estate.

Despite their middle-class careers, the values and mores of the upper-class New England society in which my family had flourished continued. My father and his brothers attended boarding school. They attended service at the Anglican Church and adopted that singular, New England, WASPish outlook on life: proper manners, few outward emotions, and so on.

After finishing boarding school, my father enrolled in and graduated from Penn State's Mont Alto Forestry School. He then spent much of his time with my grandfather, purchasing land on the cheap and reselling it for profit.

It was the land business that brought my grandfather and my father to upstate New York in the late 1960s. My father was twenty-one years old at the time. The pair arrived in a small town in northern New York State called Altona and established themselves within the town campground. This was their base of operations in the summer of 1968 as they traveled the northern counties of New York, along the Canadian border, purchasing and selling land.

Soon after setting up their base in the town park, my father drove less than a mile down Altona's main road to Stark & Guay IGA, a little country grocery store that sat in the dead center of town. My dad parked out front and went inside for supplies.

While he was in the store, Lois Stark, the daughter of one of the owners, left her parents' home next door and walked through the small parking lot to the store front. She noticed a Penn State sticker on one of the parked cars. Lois had recently obtained her master's degree from Penn State, and she walked faster up the front steps of her father's store, anxious to see who was driving the car with the school's sticker.

Lois Stark, my mother, was the only child of Halsey and Margurette Stark. Margurette's family, the Guays, comprised French Canadian immigrants (which in that area of the country meant only that at some point they moved a few miles from one side of the border to the other). The family farm was located in Champlain, New York, not far from the shores of Lake Champlain. My grandmother had six brothers and sisters.

Halsey Stark, my grandfather, was more of a townie than a farmer. He married Margurette Guay when they were both young and soon established a grocery store in the middle of Altona. At some point, Halsey caught the political bug, and he ran for and secured several town offices. After success on the town level, he decided to run for the county clerk position. Halsey won that election and held the position for twenty years.

With his dual role of businessman and politician, and with Margurette at home with their new daughter Lois, my grandfather brought a business-savvy partner on at the store: Alfreda, one of my grandmother's younger sisters. Alfreda ran the IGA until the family sold the business following Halsey's early death in 1971.

Lois was an asthmatic child, requiring frequent trips to hospitals in nearby Plattsburgh, New York, and in Montreal, Quebec. Asthma, like type 1 diabetes, is an autoimmune disease, but in those days it did not dawn on anyone that the asthma was very likely exacerbated by the cigarette smoking of both my grandparents.

Encouraged by her father, Lois excelled throughout high school. She was college bound, or rather, her father was bound and determined that his daughter would go to college and make something of herself.

Leaving a high school graduating class of thirteen, my mother enrolled at Boston University as an undergrad in 1960. Those were the days of limited options for all but the rare woman. My mother felt hers were limited to nursing or teaching. She chose teaching and became part of the university's Sargent College, where she majored in health and physical education.

After graduating from Boston University in 1964, my mother moved to Pennsylvania and attended graduate school at Penn State. Two years later, she returned home with a master's degree in health and physical education and began to look for a job in upstate New York. Then she walked into the Stark & Guay IGA in search of the driver of the car with the Penn State bumper sticker.

By all accounts, my parents hit it off almost immediately upon meeting in that little country store. They began a whirlwind romance that culminated in their marriage one year later.

After their wedding and a honeymoon trip through Quebec, my parents settled into a little house they rented in Plattsburgh, a few short blocks from my mother's new teaching job at the State University of New York at Plattsburgh and twenty miles from her parents' home. My father, at the encouragement of my mother, took advantage of this proximity to SUNY Plattsburgh and returned to school to obtain his bachelor's degree. He did so two years later, earning a degree in education that he would never use.

Following graduation, my father continued working in the land business with his father while looking for additional employment. He apparently did not have to look long or far and was quickly offered a position by the president of the local Champlain Valley Federal Savings

& Loan. My father accepted and remained with that bank for many years.

Not content with the small rented house in the city, my parents began to look for a place in the country. After some searching, they found a home six miles from the store where they had first met. The property consisted of ten acres, with two ponds, a large farmhouse, a barn, and several outbuildings. It needed a lot of work, but my parents knew it was for them. They bought the house, with help via a loan from Alfreda, thinking it would be a perfect place to raise a family.

I was born on March 10, 1972, three years after my parents' marriage and three months after the death of my mother's father, Halsey. I was a healthy baby boy, and my parents were typical first-time parents — proud, ecstatic, and scared. After a little time off following my birth, my mother returned to work. Spared from day care, I was watched during the day by a neighbor, my grandmother Margurette, or my great-aunt Alfreda while my parents were at work.

Three years after my birth, my grandmother and great-aunt stayed home with me while my mother gave birth to my brother, Jonathan Charles Beach, on June 15, 1975. Like many older siblings, I am confident that I was happy and confused at the same time, not sure what a little brother was or what it would all mean for our happy family of three.

I remember going to the hospital with my grandmother to pick up my new brother and mom and bring them home. Those were the days, after all, when mothers stayed in the hospital for a few days after giving birth and were not rushed out the door within twenty-four hours. I rode to the hospital with Grandma; Dad was in the National Guard and had been called away in a bit of unfortunate timing.

I was three years old and had missed Mom for a couple days, so I am sure my excitement was considerable. I have a dim memory of seeing my mom wheeled out to us in a wheelchair, holding a baby in her hands. I was happy.

My brother Jon was healthy for the first twenty-four months of his life, and I adjusted to our family of three plus one fairly well. While there were the routine minor eruptions of jealousy and confusion with respect to my baby brother and the attention that I now had to share with him, overall I was increasingly happy with my status as big brother.

My brother's health began to deteriorate before he reached the age of two. In the winter of 1977, my parents both noticed that Jon was having trouble crawling, often dragging one leg. He had a bright red rash on his small body, was running a fever, and appeared to be in considerable pain. After repeated trips to the pediatrician in Plattsburgh failed to resolve the problem, my parents decided to seek another opinion.

My parents took Jon across Lake Champlain via ferry to a hospital in Burlington, Vermont, and a highly recommended pediatrician. They did not know it at the time, but the ferry ride across the lake to Vermont was one that, for Jon and my mother, would become a routine, monthly trip for the next sixteen years.

Unlike the apparently confused doctor in Plattsburgh, the pediatrician who Jon saw in Burlington, Dr. James MacKay, quickly rendered a diagnosis. My baby brother had juvenile rheumatoid arthritis (JRA). JRA is a chronic form of arthritis that affects children. It is an autoimmune condition characterized by a body rash, joint paint, swollen, red joints, and limping or, in the case of a crawling child, the dragging of one leg.

Looking back, it is hard to imagine how the pediatrician in Plattsburgh missed such obvious indications. It is less difficult to see why for the rest of our respective childhoods, my parents took Jon and me across the lake to Burlington for all but the simplest health issues.

Dr. MacKay sent my parents and Jon home with an intense regimen of children's aspirin and a lot of literature on JRA. To this day, I can smell the hundreds of bottles of pink pills that we went through in those early years. Before he could chew, my mother had to crush the pink aspirin and give it to Jon that way.

The aspirin helped alleviate the rash and fever, and Jon seemed to be in less pain under the regimen. I have faint memories of being envious of the "pink treats" that my brother got so often each day.

For some time, along with the aspirin, Jon had to wear a shiny metal leg brace to help him move his leg so that it did not drag behind his body as he crawled. It was cumbersome for a baby. I don't remember ever being envious of the brace.

Within two years, my little brother's JRA was officially in remission. Jon was walking, talking, and feeling well. He was healthy and we were all happy. We spent our summers camping with my parents and playing in the woods surrounding our house. During the winters, we skated on the pond in front of our house. Our play was often interrupted with fighting, usually brought on by a good measure of sibling teasing. These squabbles were always short lived, though, and our play quickly resumed. Jon and I played, argued, and played some more. All was well, we were brothers.

Chapter Three

———～～———

SICK ANGEL

I turned seven years old in March 1979, and Jon turned four the following June. By October of that year, Jon's JRA was officially in remission, he had started preschool, and I was several weeks into second grade. I remember my teacher's face but not her name. All I really recall of second grade, and of being seven, is Christmas. Christmastime at that age is usually memorable: the new bike, new ball, and in the late 1970s, the latest *Star Wars* toys. But my Christmas memories of that year are colored a different hue.

Jon and I attended St. John's Academy. That made us "johnnies" around Plattsburgh for most of our childhood. St. John's was one of several local catholic schools. The parish was an Irish one, distinguishing it from the several French Canadian parishes in town.

My brother and I were not practicing Catholics, but we were tuition-paying students. Our lack of church attendance and our home twenty miles from the school and its surrounding neighborhoods made us unlike most of our classmates. We were not quite outcasts but were certainly apart. While it adhered to the typically strict Catholic agenda, the school attempted to make room for students like my brother and me in all aspects of the scholastic calendar.

It was in that spirit that Jon, as a preschooler, found himself cast as an angel in the St. John's Christmas pageant. Though I would join the Yuletide chorus for many a pageant in years to come, I seem to have decided to remain in the audience that year. My four-year-old brother would be the only family star for Christmas 1979. What we did not know that December was that he would remain on a different, if not elevated, stage for the rest of our lives.

The pageant was held every year during the six o'clock mass on Christmas Eve. Sister Filisitos had been running the celebrated event for years. Dressed in her blue, black, and white habit, she cut an imposing figure. The sister was at least five foot ten, had ramrod posture, and unlike most of those in her profession, had managed to stay lean, as well as mean.

Preparation for each Christmas pageant began in November, when Sister Filisitos called all interested kids to the elementary school library for singing auditions. She lined up the boys and, playing a few traditional carols on her small Casio keyboard, led what always must have been a motley bunch through the choruses.

Though reportedly deaf in one ear, no one doubted the sister's ability to wean out the least talented. With a couple of rounds of "Joy to the World" and "Silent Night," the boys who would participate in that year's pageant choir and as singing angels were selected. Those who did not make the sister's cut were told, encouragingly, that they might be chosen as a pageant character. If not one of the three wise men then certainly the position of an ass always needed filling.

The same selection process was repeated for the girls, or so we were told. Sister Filisitos always adhered to the tried and true separation of the sexes. I am confident that in her mind boys and girls singing together presented too much temptation for both groups.

In November 1979, my little brother decided to try out for the pageant. Jon not only made Sister Filisitos's cut, but he was selected for one of the most coveted roles. He would be an angel on Christmas Eve.

I am sure that upon hearing the news of my brother's pending angelic rise my mother was simultaneously thrilled and stressed. Never one to allow good tidings to wash completely over her, my mother must have immediately begun to think and rethink every impact of this announcement during the thirty or so days leading up to the big event. As always, she thought about every task that needed her attention and adhered to its every detail.

Fortunately, my memories of that Christmas are not burdened with such complications. My little brother was selected to be an angel, and a white angel costume was made, complete with gold trim and a glimmering gold halo. The Sunday afternoon that Jon obediently tried it on, there were oohs and aahs from the family members in attendance. A picture was snapped of my angelic brother in front of the Christmas tree already glowing in our living room.

A week before Christmas Eve and the annual pageant, Jon got sick. Hopes that the illness would be a twenty-four- or even forty-eight-hour bug were dashed as his symptoms continued into the fourth and fifth day. When consulted, the doctor was confident that it was just a nasty virus that had to be ridden out.

On December 23, with the pageant just twenty-four hours away, the white-and-gold angel costume was carefully folded and, together with the accompanying golden halo, placed in the bottom drawer of a dresser in my brother's bedroom. The Christmas angel was very sick.

Chapter Four

———❧———

D-Day

About a week after Christmas, my brother recovered from the virus that prevented him from assuming his role among the heavenly host. The virus was, like most, never identified, but it was nasty. Jon spent days unable to do anything other than lay in his bed, forcing down sips of ginger ale. Despite already being on the small side, he lost weight. Strangely, the virus did not spread to my parents or me. We remained healthy—my parents as comforting nurses and me as abandoned playmate.

The winter weeks that started 1980 are a blur to me, with only two events standing out: my brother's bout with the unknown virus and the day we learned of its most lasting scar. The second half of that day of discovery is carved into my gray matter forever.

January 11, 1980, started as a typical winter day in upstate New York. It was cold, and many inches of snow remained on the ground. Our house was about twenty miles from our school. That meant I had to get up around six each morning to make sure I had time to dress, eat breakfast, and brush my teeth before my dad summoned me to his car, where I rode shotgun on his commute to work.

Listening to my parents' conversation before school, I learned that my brother did not feel well for the third morning in a row. He was acting sluggish. He was cranky, an unusual disposition for him in those early years and even now. He was also very thirsty, slugging down glass after glass of water. My parents were worried. I could tell this from the slight changes in their tone that morning. Mom mentioned the Christmas virus, and Dad answered with a groan of tired anticipation. I said nothing about Jon. I just wanted to get to school.

The drive to school that day with Dad was typical. In good weather, the drive took about twenty minutes. My dad's car was plain, equipped with an AM radio that was never turned on. We rode together, as we always did, in complete silence. I killed the time by pressing my forehead against the still-frosted glass of the passenger window, feeling the numbing cold against my smooth skin, and staring out into the frozen countryside that passed by in a sixty-mile-per-hour whirl.

Twenty-five minutes after leaving our house, Dad pulled the car into the drive of St. John's Academy and I prepared to bail out—a command Dad used each morning at the end of this silent routine. Those were often the only words spoken between house and school, issued just before he remembered a rushed "good-bye." The command was given, the good-bye was spoken, and I was out of the car. With my backpack strapped to my back over my thick winter coat, I ran to the glass doors of the school that were already swinging closed from the last entry.

I have no memory of that day at school. My next memory begins at 2:30 that afternoon when school was dismissed. A lot had happened while I was in class.

~~~

Jon did get out of his bed that morning, shortly after Dad and I left on our silent ride to town. He remained unusually sluggish and grumpy though. My mom knew that she had to get into town to teach her classes and that preschool was not an option that day. Her instincts told her something was not right with Jon.

The morning's alternative to preschool came in the form of Ernie Coons, a professor of health education and fitness, like my mom, at SUNY Plattsburgh. "Uncle" Ernie, as we knew him, and his wife, "Aunt" Helene, had been my parents' best friends for several years. They lived about seven miles down the road. In fact, our house was nearly equidistant between my grandmother's house and the Coonses' home, the center of a north–south axis where much of my young life took place.

Believing, correctly, that Ernie's schedule that day was clear, my mom picked up the telephone to give him a call. Helene was a high school teacher and would be in class, but Ernie could watch Jon. Ernie answered my mom's call and quickly agreed Jon could stay at his house while my mom taught her classes. With that set, they thought the day would be fine.

Arriving at Ernie's house an hour or so after calling him that morning, my mom parked her burgundy Jeep in the driveway, got out, and opened the door for my brother. Jon adored Ernie Coons and loved the trips to his house. He was always anxious to get there, so much so that the news of pending trips to the Coonses' house was kept from my brother until the absolute last minute to avoid the trying repetition of "When are we going to Uncle Ernie's?"

That morning was different. Rather than watching Jon dash from Jeep to Ernie's front door, my mom had to peel my little brother out of the seat. His lethargy was getting worse. He was thirsty too, so very thirsty. Holding his hand, Mom walked Jon to the door and knocked. Ernie answered with a smile that noticeably faded when he saw my brother.

With my brother parked on the floor in the Coonses' family room, my mom and Ernie spoke quietly in the kitchen. Glancing through the doorway to the family room floor, Ernie told my mom he was worried about Jon. Something was not right. My mom agreed, and relayed her observations of the past two days. Jon was increasingly lethargic, and the only thing he wanted to do was drink glass after glass of water.

For Ernie, that thirst thing rang a bell. Ernie told my mom that he thought he had a few urine test strips left from a relative's visit. The relative had diabetes. My mom laughed nervously in response, thinking that my brother could not have diabetes. "It's the drinking," Ernie persisted.

Feeling there was nothing to lose, my mom agreed to let Ernie test Jon before she left for class. Ernie left the kitchen and went upstairs, returning a few minutes later carrying a small brown glass bottle, with white label and screw-top cap. There were only three or four test strips in the bottle, and they were old, but it was worth a shot.

My mom went to the living room and then took Jon back through the kitchen to an adjacent half bathroom, where Ernie stood ready with a test strip. With a bit of convincing, my brother took down his pants and started to pee into the toilet. Ernie held the test strip in the stream. My brother finished peeing.

The brown glass bottle had a color chart on its back label, ranging from dark brown to barely perceptible blue white. To test the amount of glucose spilling into the urine, one simply dipped a test strip into urine and then waited sixty seconds for the two tiny, square reaction pads on the strip's tip to turn color. The darker the color, the higher the blood sugar, and vice versa.

Ernie brought the test strip up against the back of the brown bottle, while my mom helped my brother pull up his pants. When she looked over to Ernie, his face was gray. The color on the tip of the test strip was darker, by several shades, than the darkest brown on the back of the bottle. The color in my mom's face quickly changed, matching Ernie's pallor. After a few moments of silence, Ernie and my mom agreed to wait a few minutes and try the test again, hoping that the first test strip would prove to be defective.

While they waited, my mom rummaged through her purse and found the number of Dr. MacKay, my brother's pediatrician in Burlington, Vermont. She would be ready if the second test mirrored the first.

At Ernie's beckoning, my four-year-old brother dragged himself back to the bathroom. Jon was more reluctant the second time, and quite likely confused as to why two adults were so interested in his pee. Ernie pulled a second test strip from the jar and repeated the procedure. This time though, my mom left my brother to his own devices when it came to hiking his pants back up. She immediately joined Ernie in an anxious stare at the test strip. Ernie held the strip against the back of the bottle, the tip of the strip trembling. They watched the tiny squares darken, and in a few seconds the color was again a dark brown.

Ernie ushered Jon back to his blanket on the family room floor, while my mom picked up the blue receiver of the kitchen telephone and dialed the number of Dr. MacKay's office in Burlington. After a brief conversation with the receptionist and a brief time on hold, my mom had Dr. MacKay on the line and found herself explaining my brother's situation. The doctor did not hesitate; he told my mom to get my brother into her car and drive to the hospital in Burlington. He would meet them there.

~~

St. John's elementary students were officially dismissed each day at 2:30 p.m. In second grade, the pending release loomed over the classroom beginning around 1:45. You could feel the tension in the air as the eyes of fifteen students frequented the black hands of the round, white-faced clock above the teacher's desk at the head of the room. Freedom was within reach and each of us knew it. We wanted out.

Although classes officially ended at 2:30 p.m., only the "walkers," who either were picked up by their parents or walked home, were dismissed from the premises at that time. The remaining students had to stay in the classroom until called down to their buses, usually around 2:50 p.m.

I had always been a walker, and my eyes were glued to that clock. Its black hands seemed to slow dramatically once they passed the two o'clock position. The movement between two and two thirty was a daily eternity.

When two thirty finally arrived on that winter afternoon of 1980, I rose from my desk and raced to the closet, where I found my book bag and the winter coat that, no matter how carefully I placed it in on the three-prong metal hook, was inevitably laying on the floor of the closet by the end of the day. I carried the two back to my desk. After carelessly shoving whatever papers I needed to bring home that evening into the book bag and stuffing my arms into my coat, I was off.

Students had to walk while in the school halls, so launch was delayed until we were through the exit doors. As always, I walked with a hint of run down the hall from the second-grade classroom, turned one corner, and with book bag dragging behind me, hit the crash bar of the glass door leading to the cold air of freedom with the palms of both hands. The door lurched open and I passed through, joining a few dozen schoolmates in a run across the schoolyard pavement to the parents who waited for us in a line of parked cars.

I knew something was wrong that afternoon when I did not see my mom's burgundy Jeep parked in its normal spot. She must have arrived at school about the same time each day, because the Jeep always seemed to be parked two or three cars from the head of the line of waiting parents. Apparently one or two moms (they were all moms back then) always wanted to pick up their walkers more than my mom did, because the Jeep was never first in line.

As I realized that the Jeep was not in its usual place, my cocksure run slowed first to a less positive jog and then a confused walk. My eyes scanned the line of cars for the Jeep. It was not there. I stood at the edge of the crusted snow in front of the school, just before the concrete of the sidewalk, running my eyes up and down the cars that were rapidly filling with children and beginning to pull away. Mom was not there.

The immediate concerns that accompanied that conclusion were interrupted when I heard a familiar voice calling my name. I turned my head to the left, and Dad was there, standing half outside of the driver's door of his car, which was parked at the end of the line. With my mind a bit foggy from this rapid departure from the routine, I did a double take and confirmed that it was my dad's car and that the man beckoning me with a wave and shout was indeed my dad. Something was wrong.

Instead of resuming my run, I walked cautiously down the sidewalk and past the few remaining cars with impatient moms at their wheels.

By the time I was close to his black car, Dad had sat back down behind the wheel and closed his door. The engine was running and I could tell by his face that he was not happy.

My dad had picked my brother and me up from school a few times when my mom was either away or sick. It was generally not a pleasant experience for anyone involved. Our after-school routine was shattered, and his workday was interrupted. On top of that, instead of driving home, where we were free to go outside and play, we would have to go to Dad's office at the bank. The bank was fun for about ten minutes, and then time dragged until five o'clock, the hour Dad would leave and drive us home.

Swinging my book bag off my back, I pushed the button on the chrome door handle and pulled the passenger door open. Dad greeted me with a "Hi Kiddo" as I sat down in the passenger seat and placed the book bag onto the floor between my legs.

"What's wrong with Mom?" I asked, looking at my dad. He was already glancing over his shoulder, preparing to pull the car from the curb.

"Nothing's wrong with Mom," he said in a matter-of-fact, flat tone that was more concerning for some reason than had it been filled with more emotion. Our car moved into the center of the school drive.

"Why are you here then?"

When I asked this, Dad was looking straight ahead and for the first time that afternoon, I noticed how pale and concerned his face looked.

"Your mom had to take your brother to Burlington to the hospital this afternoon."

I thought for a moment and wondered whether I had missed some conversation that morning, some clue that Jon had a doctor's appointment across the lake later in the day. I did not think I had, and I focused again on Dad's worried look.

"What's wrong with him?"

Our car pulled out of the school drive as Dad made a right onto Broad Street.

"They don't know yet."

Broad Street was busy this time of day, with four schools being dismissed within a mile of one another.

"Is he sick?"

Dad braked and stopped the car for the red light at Broad and South Catherine Streets.

"They don't know yet," he repeated.

It was clear that my dad was telling the truth. I changed my line of questioning.

"Are we going to the bank?"

"Yes."

"How long do I have to stay there?"

"Until five o'clock. Then we'll go home."

That was the first normal thing I had heard or seen for at least ten minutes. That was routine. Despite not wanting to stay at the bank for another two-and-a-half hours, I felt better.

Dad took a left onto Oak Street and the next right into the employee parking lot of the Margaret Street branch of Champlain Valley Federal Savings & Loan. That was the bank.

We parked the car in my dad's usual spot, near the chain-link fence enclosing the back of the parking lot. Leaving the car, we walked the short distance to the rear entrance of the two-story, pale-brick bank building. Walking down the back hall, we were soon in the main lobby, where the tellers still on duty said hello to me from behind the counter.

Dad's office was toward the front of the first-floor lobby, directly across from the tellers' counter. I had always liked his office. Part of the office was under the front stairs, which gave it a partially slanted ceiling and a "secret" door to a small closet. That door was smaller than me at seven years old, so it was special, and I would often open it to play within the closet's confines. The rest of the office was normal: typical ceiling, walls, desk, and chairs.

I walked into the office, following Dad, who took off his suit jacket, placed it on a hanger on the coat tree standing in the corner, sat down behind his desk, and resumed whatever work he was doing before he had left to pick me up. I took a seat in one of the smaller chairs against the wall opposite his desk. The chair was metal with burgundy vinyl seats. I put my book bag, brought from the car on dad's orders, on the floor and stared at my dad working behind the desk.

It was quiet for a minute or two. Before long, though, I began to squirm. As I shifted around in the vinyl seat, still watching my dad work, the chair began to emit a cacophony of squeals and flatulence-like noises.

Dad stopped his work and looked at me over his papers.

"Hey; sit still," he said quietly. "Find something to do."

I looked back at him and down at my book bag. It was going to be a long two hours.

After rummaging around my book bag, I did find a couple of small rubber toys that I had acquired from several trips to the family dentist. I was busy smashing the orange rubber sports car with the lime-green rubber duck when my dad's desk phone rang. He hit a button, picked up a receiver, and said "Yeah Sue?" I imagine the response to that was a curt "your wife is on the phone," because Dad said "thanks" and hit another button.

The green duck continued to smash the orange car while my parents spoke. I did not really listen, but I occasionally turned from the colliding rubbing toys to look at my dad's face while he spoke into the phone or pressed the receiver against his ear to better absorb the news from the other end of the line.

It was pretty clear, even to a seven-year-old boy, that the telephone conversation between my parents was not a good one. Dad's face was ashen, and I turned back to my stupid rubber toys when I thought I saw the glisten of a tear forming in one of his eyes. Something was very wrong with Jon.

I did not look up when Dad placed the receiver back down onto the phone's cradle. I wanted to, but I kept my head down and smashed the duck into the car a few more times. I didn't want to see Dad upset. I knew he was; I could feel it in the room.

A few minutes later, I broke the silence engulfing us.

"What's wrong with Jon?"

"You're brother has diabetes."

There it was. The answer was spoken, and the words were let out into the room. The rest of the conversation happened in less than a minute, but I will always remember each of the words—and the tears that flowed with them.

"Are they coming home now?"

"No, they have to stay in the hospital for a while."

"How long?"

"They don't know yet."

"What's dia… what's diabetes?"

"It's a disease that makes you sick."

"Will he get better?"

"No."

"It's my fault." The tears trickled down my face.

"Why do you say that?"

"Because I fight too much with him! It's my fault."

"No. No, it's not your fault. It's no one's fault."

"Are we going home soon?"

"Soon."

～～

We did leave my dad's office a bit earlier than 5:00 p.m. on that day. After stopping home and changing clothes, we drove to my grandmother's house, just six miles down the road. My mom's mother lived in the grandest house in town, a large, white, late Victorian situated in the center of the small village. My grandfather had died the Christmas Eve before I was born. My grandmother never remarried, nor am I aware of male company in her life since my birth. Instead, she lived in that large house with her sister, Alfreda.

Knocking was not something my family did before entering my grandmother's house, a long-standing custom that my brother pays the price for today as he lives there now. I am sure that Dad did not knock before he entered that cold January night in 1980. We found Grandma and Auntie sitting in the family room. Grandma was sitting in a green, faux leather recliner — a place she had, apparently, inherited from her late husband. Auntie was sitting on the nearby couch. Both were watching television and greeted us with sincere delight, as they always did.

Grandma and Auntie knew that Mom had taken Jon to the hospital in Burlington, and they were anxious to hear my dad's news. I sat on the floor and listened as Dad relayed the diagnosis to them. I still had no idea what diabetes was or what it would mean for my family, but hearing my dad's voice and watching my grandmother's and aunt's reactions, I knew it was not good.

Dad tried his best to answer Grandma's many questions. In reality, he only knew what little Mom had been able to convey during their short telephone conversation that afternoon in the office and another brief call later at home. I did not understand then that adults could be as clueless as children, but we were all in the dark when it came to diabetes.

After stating that he would be going to the hospital the next day and securing Auntie's agreement to pick me up after school, Dad excused himself and went to the kitchen to get some water. With his departure, the room fell silent.

For some reason, the silence was worse than anything else, and I began to cry. Grandma beckoned me to her, and I rose off the floor and walked over to the arm of the green chair. She put her arm around me and reassured me that everything was going to be okay. Her words were comforting, and I craved her nearness. I wanted my tears to stop. I wanted to be a big boy. It was so confusing and sounded so bad. I knew it was my fault.

"Grandma, it's my fault isn't it?"

"You mean your brother being sick?" she asked softly.

"Yeah."

"Randall don't you ever say that again. It's not your fault; it's no one's fault. Sometimes these things just happen." Her voice was still soft, but it was also firm. She wanted me to know her words were true—a command, rather than a request.

"Okay, Randall? Do you understand what I am saying?"

I hesitantly nodded my head in agreement, wiping some tears away with the back of my hand.

"Good. Your brother's going to be okay. You'll see." She sounded very confident, surely more confident than she actually was.

I shrugged, still unsure, but said, "Okay Grandma."

After returning home from Grandma's house, it was bedtime. I put on my pajamas and got under the covers. Dad came in and told me a story. My dad would make up stories about me and my brother and things we had done during the day. I loved that much more than when he would read from a book. His made-up stories were special and all about Jon and me. But Dad read from a book that night. The events of that day had been nightmarish and were surely not suitable for bedtime stories.

With the lights off and my door half shut, I lay in my bed and started to cry. It didn't matter what my dad and grandmother had said. I knew that diabetes, whatever it was, was my fault. My brother was sick in the hospital and it was my fault.

Chapter Five

―❦―

FIRST VISIT

Two days after Jon's diagnosis, I was allowed to travel with Dad across Lake Champlain to Burlington, Vermont, to visit my little brother in the hospital. It was also a trip for me to see my mom. She had not left Jon's side since the diagnosis. She spent the nights sleeping in my brother's hospital room on a cot the hospital provided for her.

I was excited to see both my brother and my mom that afternoon, and school seemed to go even slower than normal. When the walkers were dismissed, I hurried to my dad's waiting car, already more familiar in the pickup line. I pulled the car door open, intending to quickly jump in, and was surprised to see Uncle Ernie in the front passenger seat next to Dad, with Aunt Helene behind them. I was happy to see the extra passengers, though, and did not mind moving to the backseat where Aunt Helene was. I opened the rear door, jumped onto wide black bench seat, closed the door, and we were off.

The ferry landing was less than ten miles from school, but that was enough time for my excitement and fear to combine unpleasantly in my gut. I don't remember the exact moment of the accident, but it happened before we got onto the ferry. I do distinctly remember walking with Dad to the garbage barrel at the ferry landing and watching as Dad threw what had been a good pair of *Star Wars* underwear into the trash.

The ferry arrived from the Vermont side a little after we had disposed of my soiled underpants. On future trips, I would spend the time waiting for the ferry's arrival skipping flat rocks across the shallows at the rocky beach, which lay beyond the paved parking lot where cars waited for the boat. I think that spot is where my dad taught me how to skip stones on water. It was a wonderful, addicting sport and one in which Dad seemed to have been a gold medalist.

Lake Champlain is a 125-mile-long body of water separating New York and Vermont and extending into southern Quebec. It is one of the largest lakes in the United States but largely unknown except to the residents of northern New York and Vermont. Some fourteen miles at its widest and boasting four hundred-foot depths, the lake can be formidable.

Two large bridges and three ferry systems link New York and Vermont across Lake Champlain. For my family, our choices were the Rouses Point Bridge, about thirty minutes north of us, or the Lake Champlain Transportation Company's ferry at Cumberland Head, a peninsula jutting into the lake just north of Plattsburgh. The ferry landing was about seventeen miles from our house, which generally made the crossing a faster route to Burlington.

In the years ahead, my parents would spend thousands of dollars crossing Lake Champlain, carting my brother back and forth between doctor appointments and hospital stays. Managing the ferry schedules would become routine. What did not become routine, and thus became the source of harrowing tales, were the few times each year when Lake Champlain reared its ugly head and presented ferry passengers with more sea than they had bargained for. At times waves can swell to four feet or more, driving the flat-bottomed ferry boat up and down their crests and troughs. Cars parked toward the bow get the extra feature of a free car wash, courtesy of Lake Champlain, as huge walls of water crash over the ferry's bow and over several rows of vehicles. On such occasions, the ferry ride is not for the faint of heart.

Driving onto the ferry that afternoon, there were no white crests in sight. The lake appeared calm and even welcoming. The deckhand directed my dad's car ahead and to the left. As soon as Dad turned the ignition key to shut the engine off, I began to get restless in the backseat.

All of the ferry boats had upper decks where passengers could sit and take in the views of the Adirondacks and Green Mountains as the boat traveled to the other side of the lake. The decks were both covered and uncovered, accommodating visitors in any type of weather. They also were equipped with a few of those gleaming silver binocular stands that beckon all children. For a mere quarter, those oval viewing stations promised to increase your view for a minute or two.

I wanted out of the car and onto the upper deck. Dad sensed my anxiousness, looked back, and told me to sit still. He assured me that we could all get out and go up as soon as the boat left the dock. Aunt Helene put her hand on my shoulder and smiled. Everyone was accommodating and kind. That was both reassuring and disturbing to me. I needed the kindness, but getting so much, especially after just wiping out my underpants, meant things were still not right. This thing with my little brother, this diabetes, was serious. I could tell.

When the last car was loaded, the deckhands pulled the heavy ropes from their ties on shore and raised the vehicle ramp. Our car was parked

in the middle of the left deck, far from any excitement that might be-
fall those cars parked in the bow, where they were separated from the
open water by two chains strung from one side of the boat to the other.
Being in the middle of the boat meant that we were close to the stairs
leading to the upper deck. I began to get squirmy again.

With the vehicle ramp secured, I felt the boat's engines rumble beneath
us. Slowly, the ferry began to move forward, away from the wood pil-
ings and the New York shore. We were off to Vermont. It was time to
get out and go outside!

True to his word, Dad looked back, smiled, and teasingly asked me if I
wanted to go upstairs. I fell for the tease, as I always did in those days.

"Yes! Please, can we go? Can we go?" I asked, bouncing up and down
on the backseat.

Perhaps I felt freer without underpants. Aunt Helene was laughing and
Dad was smiling. I could almost feel Uncle Ernie's grin through the
back of his head. For a brief moment, no one would have guessed the
passengers in our car were headed to the hospital to visit a very sick
four-year-old boy.

"I suppose we can," Dad said, still smiling. "Ernie, you coming?"

The answer was the opening of his door. Uncle Ernie was coming.

"How about you Helene?" my dad asked as he pulled the handle on
his own door.

"No, it's too windy," she responded. "You guys go ahead."

By the time I heard Aunt Helene say no, my hands were on the door
handle on my side of the backseat and I was pushing the door open. I

wanted out and up. Luckily, traffic had been light and the deckhand had made sure there was lots of room between the rows of cars that day, because my car door swung wildly and would surely have hit the side of the car parked next to us had it been closer.

"Easy!" I heard Dad command as he walked around the rear of our car and grabbed my hand. He closed my door for me and, placing his hand on my shoulder, gently pushed me toward the metal stairs just to the right of the car whose side I might have swiped. I fixed my eyes on the stairway as I was guided ahead and saw the back of Uncle Ernie's head just before it disappeared up the stairs. Apparently, I was not the only one anxious to get on deck.

Dad and I walked up the steep metal stairway and onto the upper deck of the ferry boat. It was a sunny day, but Aunt Helene was right about the wind. Our hair began to blow back as we took the final step up and planted our feet onto the steel upper deck. I saw Uncle Ernie leaning against the solid steel side of the ferry, looking out over the water. I ran across the deck and joined him there.

The side of the deck was fairly high, and I could just see over it if I stood on my tippy-toes. I strained to peer over the steel and saw the blue of the surrounding lake. Reaching down, Uncle Ernie grabbed me by the waist and boosted me up. With the added height, I saw for miles. I focused on the waves of blue and the white froth created by the ferry's travels through the water. I wondered what kind of fish were beneath us and whether Champ, the legendary Lake Champlain monster, was near.

Dad joined us on the rail and added his hand to my waist. I was held and secure. The wind blew in our faces, but I did not care. I was happy with my view from above.

Looking ahead, I could see the Vermont shore getting closer. The

Cumberland Head ferry traveled between Plattsburgh and Grand Isle, Vermont. Grand Isle is one of several large, inhabited islands on the lake and is connected to the Vermont mainland via a causeway. As much as I wanted to see Mom and Jon that day, I was happy riding on top of the ferry boat, held tight by Dad and Uncle Ernie. It was disappointing to feel the boat turning toward its Vermont landing.

When the sound of the powerful engines lessened, signaling that the boat was slowing down and preparing to dock, Dad declared it was time to go back to the car. Uncle Ernie and Dad lowered me down from the side, and the three of us walked across the deck to the stairs. Uncle Ernie went down first, then me, and then Dad. In another minute we were loaded back in the car, joining Aunt Helene, who had been reading a magazine she had brought from home. The engines rumbled beneath us and the car vibrated along with the entire vehicle deck as the captain effortlessly slipped the big boat into its docking berth and reversed the engines for last-minute maneuvers and to slow the boat's momentum.

Next came the clanking of steel against steel as the deckhands unhooked the two bow chains and dragged them across the deck to their unloading position. As the vehicle ramp was lowered from the shore, Dad turned the key in the ignition and our own engine came to life. The deckhand stood at the bow and signaled to the lead car in the row to our left to proceed ahead. I watched as each car passed us and drove off the boat. With that row complete, it was our turn.

Dad shifted our car into drive and waited for the car ahead of us to move forward. Within no time, we were off the ferry deck and onto Vermont pavement. Our next stop would be the parking lot of the hospital.

It takes about thirty minutes to drive from the Grand Isle ferry landing to Burlington. The roads are mostly country roads, winding through the Champlain islands and the mainland until hitting Interstate 89. We took the first exit for Burlington and a few minutes later were parking in the large lot adjacent to the hospital. Mom had given Dad directions into the hospital lobby to the correct bank of elevators, and he led our little group there without incident.

My little brother was in the pediatric wing of the hospital. When the elevator chimed its arrival, the door opened and we poured into the car. Uncle Ernie pressed the button for the fourth floor.

We were all anxious to see Jon. Despite our frequent arguments, and even though I sometimes picked on my little brother, I had missed playing with him after school. More than that, though, I wanted to see him with my own eyes to make sure that he was still there. I needed to know that Jon still existed and was going to come back home. It had only been a few days, but to my seven-year-old mind those days had been weeks.

In addition to Jon, I was anxious to see Mom. Being without a little brother for a few days was bad, but being without a mom was worse. Grandma and Auntie always made sure I was taken care of and fed well, and Dad tried his best to keep me happy, but they were not adequate substitutes for Mom. I had spoken to my mom on the telephone a couple of times since she had been stationed by my brother's side in Burlington, but it wasn't enough. I needed my mom. I wanted her back.

When the bell chimed again, the door to the elevator slid open and we were on the fourth floor. The four of us stepped onto the white tile of the pediatric wing and were immediately confronted with the imposing nursing station. I stood a little behind Dad, brushing up against the gift-wrapped present he had brought for my brother, as he walked toward the counter where a nurse sat speaking on the phone.

Glancing up at us, the nurse hastened a few last words into the telephone receiver and then placed the handset back onto its cradle. She smiled and winked at me.

"Good afternoon folks," the nurse said with a surprising amount of cheer evident in her voice. "Who are you here to see?"

"Jonathan Beach," Dad answered for us all.

"Oh, I should have known!" was the cheerful nurse's reply. I'm not sure that any of the adults questioned this response. Why she should have known did not occur to me.

"My name is Helen," the nurse said, standing and extending her hand to my dad. "You're Jonathan's father, I bet."

"Yes, Randy Beach," Dad responded, taking Helen's hand gingerly.

"He is going to be so happy to see you all!" Helen said, smiling wide and turning out of her chair. She walked around the counter to the front and stopped.

"And I bet you are Randall," the smiling nurse said to me as she stooped down, hands cupping her knees, to bring her smile closer to me.

I turned shyly away, pressing closer to my dad. Helen did not miss a beat though, and she was quickly erect and ushering us to follow her down the hall. Dad brought me out from against his leg and pushed me out in front of him as we dutifully trailed Helen.

Unlike the walls surrounding the fourth-floor nurse's station and most of the other walls of the hospital, the walls in the halls of the pediatric wing were not stark white. Instead, they were covered with various murals. Some sections had paintings of Bugs Bunny and other cartoon characters in scenes of mischief and fun. Other sections of the walls had jungle scenes with monkeys and the like. It still looked like a hospital hall, just not as serious.

Helen stopped in front of a doorway halfway down the hall from the nurse's station, and our group stopped behind her. She knocked on the jam of the open door and announced that my brother had "special visitors." We did not have to wait long for an answer. Mom popped her head out of the doorway and surveyed our group. Finding that it was us, the rest of her body followed her head as she stepped out of the room and into the hall.

Once in the hall, Mom greeted us all brightly and made sure we were all introduced to Helen, whom we quickly learned was my brother's favorite nurse. We later learned that this favoritism ran both ways as Helen expressed a clear preference and love for my brother.

With those introductions, Mom ushered us into the room. Surprisingly, Helen stayed with our group. My brother was sitting up in his bed playing with a few Matchbox cars when we entered his room. It was only partially his room; we would meet another boy and his mother across the pulled-back curtain before we left later that evening.

Jon's face lit up when he saw our group walking into the room. He jumped from sitting to standing on the bed and gave first my dad then each of the adults a big hug. He was laughing and smiling when I touched his arm, and I smiled with him. I was genuinely happy to see my little brother that afternoon.

After the initial greetings, my brother was presented with first my dad's gift, a box that when unwrapped revealed a Pink Panther doll. The mischievous Pink Panther was my brother's favorite cartoon character at the time. Uncle Ernie also produced a wrapped present for my brother. Jon ripped the gift wrap off in no time to reveal a John Deere farm tractor. Jon's face was one big smile, and everyone on our side of the room was laughing and smiling with him. All was good.

We stayed at the hospital for several hours on that first visit. We all watched as the nurse came in before dinner was served to test my brother's blood sugar and give him a shot of insulin. Jon went with the nurse into the bathroom for the urine test and was given the shot in his leg when he came back.

I was not surprised to hear Jon cry when the nurse put the needle into his leg and pushed the plunger. It looked like it hurt to me. Mom explained that this would be our way of life for now on: urine tests and insulin shots. I asked whether a nurse was going to be coming home with us. This triggered nervous laughter from the adults in the room.

Mom then explained to me that she was learning how to give Jon the shots and that Dad would learn too. Someday, she said, Jon will give them to himself. I looked at Jon, who was back on the bed playing with his new tractor. It seemed doubtful to me that my little brother would willingly stab himself with a needle. That was something adults did to children, not an act that children took upon themselves.

"When can I give him a shot?" I asked Mom, still watching my brother playing on the bed. Perhaps this diabetes was not so bad after all. Pricking my brother with a needle might even be fun on some days.

Mom did not seem quite prepared for that question.

"Well, we will see," was the best she managed to get out. "If you want to learn, I am sure you can once your dad and I get good at doing it ourselves.

I did not know it at the time, but Mom's hesitant response that day was the diabetes door partially shutting on me. While I learned many things about diabetes and how to help my little brother, I never learned how to give my brother a shot and don't recall that such training was ever offered to me. On that day, though, Mom's answer satisfied me. I would learn about the shots and this diabetes thing too. Everything seemed okay.

Time passed, and then the cafeteria staff brought a tray of food into Jon's room and set up the table over his bed. My brother could not leave the pediatric wing and did not seem to mind. I was a bit jealous of the novelty of dinner in bed but felt better when all of the adults and I went down to the hospital cafeteria. It served hot dogs.

As the adults around me listened to Mom tell stories of her last few days at the hospital and discuss more details about the diagnosis, I ate my hot dog and watched the other cafeteria diners. Most were in some sort of nurse's or doctor's uniform, but I did see a few other families like ours. I wondered which members of their families were missing from the table and enjoying the luxury of dinner in bed.

After dinner, we all returned to my brother's room on the fourth floor. We sat around the bed for a while longer, talking about what my brother ate for dinner and about his adventures on the pediatric wing. It seemed that Jon had taken a liking not only to Nurse Helen but also to several of the doctors performing rounds on the floor. This affection had become mutual, and the day before Jon had joined one of the young doctors on his rounds, visiting each patient in the ward. This tale amused the adults around me. It seemed that my brother was having a pretty good time in the hospital.

My initial concern for Jon was wearing off the more we stayed around him and the hospital. He was fine. He looked okay. He had presents and toys, was served his meals in bed, and played with the doctors and nurses. On top of all that, Jon got to stay with Mom while I had to stay with Dad and go to school. Something did not seem fair already. I was not liking this diabetes thing.

Luckily for me, just as my internal questioning and impatience were on the rise, Dad announced that we had better get going back home. For the first time during our visit, I noticed my brother's smile fade as Dad's words filled the room. I could see his disappointment and I looked away. I was ready to go.

We all said good-bye to Jon and pledged that we would return soon. Mom announced that she would walk us out to the parking lot. Jon turned his attention back to playing with his new toys, and the rest of us left the room and walked to the elevators.

Mom went down to the hospital lobby with us. She and Dad talked about the coming days and our respective school and work schedules. They agreed that if Jon was not released from the hospital by Friday, Dad and I would come back to visit Saturday morning.

Mom stopped in the glass vestibule that contained all of the automatic sliding glass doors that were so fascinating to me. The adults said their good-byes and Mom bent down and hugged me. Tears began to flow down my cheeks. I missed my mom, and I wanted her to come home with us. I asked her if she would, and she assured me she would be back soon. She had to stay with Jon. I understood.

On the way to the car, my dad picked me up and carried me on his shoulders. The air was cool against my wet cheeks, but I was glad to be up high and glad to be with my dad. We found our car and piled back in.

Dad drove through the maze of the parking lot and around to the front of hospital. Mom was still standing in the glass vestibule, waving to us. Dad did not stop, but I jumped up onto the backseat, waving frantically to Mom. As we turned out into the drive, I continued to wave at her through the rear window until her form was only a blur. That singular moment has not left me in more than thirty years.

Chapter Six

THE TRANSFORMED HOUSE

Jon and my mom returned home from that initial hospital stay after about a week. Mom spent the next weeks reorganizing our house and meeting with my brother's teachers and school officials. Everything was changing within our family, and changing quickly.

Our household transformed in some fundamental ways. My brother now had a drawer in the laundry room, just off the kitchen, devoted to him. This might not seem like a big change, but until then the laundry and the kitchen were the exclusive domain of my mom, and their drawers and cupboards were filled only with foodstuffs and kitchen and laundry equipment. Now, Jon had his own space in those rooms. Yes it was filled with such unpleasantries as needles and test strips, but it was still his. My dad did not have such a dedicated space. I certainly did not.

Another big change was our family diet, including the immediate introduction of soda into our household. Before Jon's diagnosis, soda was not found in our house. We drank juice — apple juice, orange juice, and grape juice especially. The introduction of diabetes into our family turned that paradigm on its head.

Juice, my mom informed me, was full of sugar, and sugar was something my brother could not have. As a result, virtually overnight we went from juice-drinking kids to soda kids. Not just any soda, mind you, diet soda. In those early days, that meant we had a choice between Tab and Fresca. This kick-started my diet soda habit that continued for decades.

Along with juice, all other sugary substances suddenly vanished from our regular diet. While we had never been junk food aficionados and ate rather healthily at home, we did enjoy our nightly desserts. Now, just as juice became diet soda, dessert morphed into fresh fruit. Cakes, brownies, pies, cookies — those items were all gone. Fruit now ruled our days and evenings.

Another significant dietary change, one willingly embraced by my brother and me, was our new ability to snack. Before diagnosis day, Jon and I were generally prohibited from snacking between meals. Mom strictly adhered to three square meals a day. Looking back, that program worked pretty well for us and for everyone else I knew. There certainly were fewer obese kids.

Diabetes brought snacks into our life. We were now permitted, even encouraged, to snack between our meals and even before bed. English muffins and peanut butter, Jell-O, nuts, fruit, and so on were made continually available to my brother and me. Each of my brother's days ended with a celebrated night snack. In the interest of fairness, I was allowed to enjoy a night snack along with Jon. The tyranny of three square meals had been vanquished by diabetes.

It was not all bliss when it came to food and diabetes, because sugar was now the official public enemy number one. That "public" qualifier is important. While sugary desserts and snacks were banned from my brother's diet, and therefore the rest of the family's, they did not disappear entirely. Instead, a Prohibition-era speakeasy system took root within our household. There were always sweet things to be found if you knew where and when to look.

Most often the forbidden desserts were found on the sideboard in the dining room. The dining room was a formal room and, as in many houses, shut off from the rest of the everyday living space until needed. In addition, there was usually a package of Oreos or Fig Newtons high on a pantry shelf intended for my dad's brown bag lunches and the occasional snack.

The rule was that sweets could come out only when my brother was either in bed or out of the house. Because he was in bed more often than he was out of the house in those days, most of the sugary substances were ingested by Dad and me in the evening after Jon's bedtime. Still, bedtime was not failsafe for our sugar cheating. I remember several instances when, watching television with Dad in the den, we had to slide our plates of cake or brownies under the couch or the nearest cover when my brother's voice and footsteps were heard from the kitchen next door. We became adept at hiding our stubborn refusal to rid our diet of sweets.

The other place of sugary refuge was my grandmother's house. As Grandma lived only six miles down the road, it was common for me to be at her house without my brother several times a week and almost every weekend. At times, these visits were overnight, but many were for thirty minutes or less. In addition to including homemade pies, cake, or pudding with any meals that were not shared with Jon, Grandma established a well-stocked supply of candy in the drawer of one of her dining room cupboards. The left-hand drawer of the large, pine cupboard became home to a seemingly endless supply of candy bars. It was usually my first stop after walking into that house. Everything is sweeter once denied.

All of this created a bifurcated food culture within our family. When my brother was present, everything was healthy and sugar-free. In his absence, Dad and I raced to the hidden sweets and gorged ourselves on the forbidden fruit. Of course, it was not fruit, and that was the point.

Along with these dietary adjustments came many changes to our family routine. Now, before each breakfast and dinner, my mom would summon my brother for his insulin shot. He would run from wherever he might be when called and take a syringe from his laundry room drawer. Mom would then remove two insulin bottles, each containing a different type of insulin, from the small shelf dedicated to diabetes in the door of the refrigerator and draw the proper mixture of insulin into the syringe.

Once the syringe was loaded, my mom and brother would agree on the location on his small body where that particular shot would be given. Mom then would pinch Jon's skin, insert the needle, and inject the insulin into my brother's body. For a long time, my four-year-old brother would cry after each shot. I can only imagine how hard it was for Mom to call Jon before each meal and listen to him cry each time.

To keep track of where Jon received his daily shots, and to ensure that a bodily location was not overused, my mom created a paper effigy of my brother. She obtained a long roll of paper like the kind the nurse unrolls over the examining table with each new patient. A good length of that paper was cut and spread flat on the floor. My brother would then lie down on his back over the paper, and my mom would playfully trace the silhouette of his body. The two of them would then circle the six possible insulin shot targets on my brother's one-dimensional likeness; each thigh, each arm, his stomach, and his bottom.

The sheet of paper with flat Jon and the marked insulin targets was then taped to a wall or door—usually in the laundry room. An *X* or a dot was placed by my brother in each target area when a shot was received in the corresponding body part. In this way, overuse of an arm, leg, or other area was avoided, and a healthy shot rotation was achieved. Each paper image of my brother's body lasted only a couple of weeks. After that, there were too many *X*s and dots covering the target zones, and a new effigy was made.

Jon's silhouette became the new record of development in our house. It replaced the penciled-in height marks that once adorned the white casing of the door leading to the basement and now would only reveal how the earlier bout with JRA was stunting Jon's growth. Those growth marks had been recorded for both of us, but now the only record was of Jon.

My brother's bathroom routine also changed in a public way. His days of peeing without notice were gone. At that time, the only way to measure blood sugar at home was via urine test strips. In reality, the urine test only gave an indication of how much glucose was in my brother's urine. Compared to the modern blood sugar monitors of today, the urine test was very inaccurate.

Nonetheless, Jon needed to test his sugar throughout each day. Mom would remind him of this constantly and escort him into the bathroom when he had to go or when he had to test. He would then pee into a plastic jug made for that purpose and a test strip would be dipped into the warm urine. We learned that, once dipped, it took sixty seconds for the results to fully appear on the test strip. There was an analog stopwatch placed in the bathroom for the countdown. Sometimes, when I was lucky, I got to run this stopwatch and announce that time was up.

If you were around Jon, you knew when he had to pee. With diabetes, discretion was out the window even when it came to the most personal acts.

Chapter Seven

REACTIONS

The most traumatic change in routine for our family was the seemingly daily interruption of our lives by the insulin reaction. The insulin reaction, or just "reaction" as it became known in our house, could come at any time during the day or night. It could sneak up on us under the cover of naptime or spring upon us during a swim or play outside. The reaction brought cries of terror into our family routine and a knot in my stomach that I can still feel so many years later.

The insulin reaction, Mom explained to me during those first few weeks, was my brother's body reacting to too much insulin and not enough blood sugar in its system. Apparently, without enough blood sugar to process, insulin became angry and made my brother's body go haywire.

In those early days, it seemed that most of Jon's reactions came during his sleep, whether that sleep was part of a daytime nap or in the middle of the night. That meant that my brother went to sleep and at some point woke up screaming and shaking. This was an unpleasant experience regardless of whether it was during the day or night. It made me wary of my brother anytime I found him asleep. I wanted him up and active, not in a sleep that might bring forth that terrible screaming and shaking.

The typical sleep-time reaction went like this. Jon would lay down for his afternoon nap. I might be taking a nap too, but being three years older, I was more likely to be reading or playing by myself. There might be thirty minutes of silence from my brother's room; I don't remember Jon snoring back then. A bloodcurdling scream would abruptly break the sleepy silence. Mom would rush up to my brother's room, with me trailing behind. I always seemed to run to the screaming, although so much of me wanted to run from it.

When we entered my brother's bedroom, Jon would almost always be sitting up in his bed, crying and screaming. His body shook uncontrollably, and his eyes, if opened, looked around his bedroom unseeing.

The cure for the reaction was the rapid introduction of glucose into my brother's body. This came in the form of sugary substances. Honey was the most common medium. My parents used to purchase wholesale boxes of small plastic packets of honey and carry those packets everywhere we went. They were in the glove box of the car, my mom's purses, my dad's briefcase, and all around the house.

Administering the honey to Jon often proved more challenging than locating it. Trying to get a trembling, screaming boy to voluntarily suck down a few packets of sweet and sticky honey was nearly impossible. This meant that Mom would have to apply the honey manually; that is, she would stick some honey on her fingers and then plunge them into my brother's mouth and rub the honey on the inside of his cheeks. This proved to be an effective technique, but it was not without its hazards. On more than several occasions, my brother clamped his teeth down on my mom's sticky, sweet fingers.

Orange juice was often the second and less perilous antidote. The glucose in the honey was quickly absorbed through my brother's cheek cells, and the violence of his body would decrease in turn. In a few minutes, my brother would become more sleepy and slower than trembling and loud. He could hold a honey packet in his hands and push its contents into his mouth himself. Once he was in this state, a glass of orange juice could be held before him and with a bit of urging, he would drink.

After a few more minutes of the juice-and-honey diet, my brother's eyes would be open and alert, and his body would be back to its normal, boyish maneuvers. This signaled the third phase of the reaction remedy — real food. Toast was often the next food fed to Jon. This was always the case for night reactions. I know that well, because I was the official toast maker for such events. The toast was adorned with a layer of butter followed by a generous spread of jam or jelly. Daytime reactions were often followed by a more elaborate snack, in which case I was out of the toast-making job.

The fourth and final stage of the reaction took hold when Jon was about halfway finished with his postreaction snack. At this point, his eyes were bright and his smile wide. He returned to his normal, laughing self with little to no recollection of the past fifteen minutes. If it was the middle of the night, he would quickly finish the toast, lie back down in bed, and instantly regain the solace of sleep. The end of a daytime reaction would bring my brother back to whatever activity he was pursuing before the event.

Jon moved on from the typical insulin reaction as if nothing had happened. This is a blessing for those inflicted with the disease and the chaos it inflicts on the body. The people surrounding the inflicted are not so lucky. While my brother resumed his slumber immediately after the nighttime reaction, my parents and I would have difficulty falling back asleep. Dad would often spend much of his valuable remaining sleep time sick to his stomach as a result of getting up so quickly from a sound sleep. Our tired and drawn faces the next morning were visible proof of the night's terror.

Daytime reactions were equally disruptive. The interrupted activity was never quite the same when resumed. Thousand-yard stares from my parents and me were not uncommon during the hours following such an event.

That was how the typical insulin reaction went for my brother and our family. They became, for me, at once routine and terrifying. Watching my little brother scream and shake uncontrollably was something I came to anticipate but never got used to. Yet, the typical was, as is so often the case, not the worst.

More severe insulin reactions were, thankfully, rare. They usually began during Jon's sleep. Occurring when my brother's blood sugar dropped to super low levels, these reactions made the typical insulin reaction look like the proverbial walk in the park.

The beginning of these severe insulin reactions was similar to any of the countless night reactions that my brother experienced throughout our childhood: a deep sleep pierced by screams of terror. Despite this initial similarity, the scene that I arrived to in my brother's bedroom during a severe reaction was different by many degrees. The tremors that shook Jon's small body were more powerful and his eyes were glued shut. The screams were not necessarily louder, but they were markedly different. The screams were more terrible, as if the well that my brother's conscience was falling into was fathoms deeper. Even the air in the room felt different during these episodes. I think we all could feel it as soon as we entered Jon's bedroom.

The departure from the norm was rapid. It was visible and unforgettable. Those terror-filled screams would stop. My brother's eyes would suddenly come unglued and open just enough that we could watch as his eyes rolled back into his head. Simultaneously, the tremors turned to full-fledge flailing. A powerful seizure overcame my little brother.

The ubiquitous honey packets were useless in the face of the seizure that racked Jon's body. My parents moved with lightning speed as I either sunk against a bedroom wall or, if I was lucky, silently slipped outside into the hallway to wait until the worst was over. Either Dad or Mom would hold Jon down against the bed to ensure that he did not hurt himself. The other would quickly leave the room and go into the bathroom next door. In the bathroom closet, on the highest of the shelves, was the remedy for such seizures: a syringe prepared with a generous helping of glucagon.

Glucagon, I later learned, is a hormone produced by the pancreas — the organ that fails all diabetics. It is the antithesis of insulin. Insulin lowers blood sugar. Glucagon raises blood sugar. Together they are the yin and yang of the pancreas's secretions.

The parent who retrieved the glucagon would reenter my brother's bedroom without a pause and, while commanding the parent holding Jon down to keep him still, inject the glucagon into my brother's writhing body. The effect was nearly instantaneous. In place of the slower recovery from less severe reactions, my brother's seizure ended in just a few seconds. His eyes would return to their normal position and begin to focus as his brain became aware again. That was my cue to go downstairs and start the toast.

When I was very young, I would cheer for the glucagon. It was so much quicker than the honey – orange juice combination. One quick dose and my brother was on the comeback. My parents, however, hated to use what I heralded as a miracle drug. Instead of praising the glucagon, they cursed it as a necessary evil. They understood the side effects.

Glucagon, though miraculous in my young eyes, was not without significant costs to the body it was injected into. The hormone causes the liver to break down fat stores into glucose. It goes to work quickly, and the glucose is rapidly released into the bloodstream. This works well and is what would happen if Jon were to be left unattended during an insulin reaction: eventually his liver would kick in and save the day.

The savior turned out to have a dark side. The injection of glucagon would rapidly pull my brother out of the seizure and raise his severely low blood sugar, but it would also make him very sick for the next day or so. He would be nauseous, vomiting many times.

It was a nasty price to pay for remedying super low blood sugar levels. These were reactions that Jon did not walk away from smiling or follow by simply rolling over into a sound sleep. He suffered through the side effects each time the magic solution was pushed into his body. My parents suffered too.

As usual, my mom suffered the most alongside my brother. My dad would be off the next morning to the refuge of his office, and I would be in school. It was Mom who had to cancel her classes for the day to stay home with Jon while he lay on his bed or the downstairs' couch, unable to keep food or water down. A diabetic who can't keep anything down is a diabetic in trouble. Diabetes played nasty games with my brother's body. The disease was, and remains, a formidable foe.

These were the reactions that I grew up around: the horrible ones with seizures and the just plain terrible ones. I quickly became suspicious of any daytime sleep that my brother might attempt. On many days, I would fight with Mom to let Jon play with me longer rather than enforce the afternoon naptime his young age demanded. I was afraid of his naps. I did not want the afternoon to be interrupted with his screams. I did not want to have to hold my trembling, screaming brother while Mom shoved globs of honey into his mouth. I did not want to be the young helper during those moments. I wanted to run away and hide.

As time went on, bedtime did not bother me as much as naptime. By the end of the day, I was tired, and once I decided to stay in my bed, I fell asleep rather easily. My own tiredness overcame the anxiety that came with the realization that my brother would also be sleeping down the hall. Nighttime also meant that Dad was home. If Jon awoke screaming, Dad would be there with Mom. At night, I was the third wheel — the toast maker. In time, I learned to make excellent toast.

Despite becoming adept at managing his diabetes, my brother had a few insulin reactions that were so spectacularly bad that they remain blazed in my memory some thirty years later. These were times that for one reason or another scared me more than others. One such reaction occurred on the Massachusetts Turnpike.

After living with diabetes for three years, my seven-year-old brother had been lucky enough to find the camp run by the Joslin Diabetes Center. The camp is located in Charlton, Massachusetts, outside of Worchester, and is considered the best diabetes camp in the world. It was a boys-only camp, staffed with diabetics, nurses, doctors, nutritionists, and other clinical experts. The camp is located on a beautiful piece of property that includes top-notch cabins, a dining facility, its own lake, a radio station, and a well-equipped infirmary. Camp Joslin is first rate, and my brother quickly learned to love it there, spending two to eight weeks there each summer as a camper, counselor in training, and then counselor, from age seven to twenty.

The Mass Pike reaction, as I have dubbed it, occurred the summer that my brother turned eleven. I was a fourteen-year-old big shot—in my own mind. Though most years my parents wisely planned for me to be at either a basketball or a soccer camp while Jon was at Camp Joslin, that particular year I found myself visiting my little brother at Camp Joslin with my mom.

We sprung my brother from camp for a day, and Mom took Jon and me to Boston. It was about an hour's ride with traffic, and we made a good day of it, visiting the New England Aquarium and later the Boston Science Museum. It was on the way back to Camp Joslin that all hell broke loose.

Despite my attempts to keep Jon awake in the car, he was tired after our busy day in Boston. Jon fell asleep in the backseat within fifteen minutes of our departure from the city. I was in the front seat, listening to some pop channel on the radio that I purposely kept turning up in hopes of waking my brother. Mom, more optimistic than me when it came to my brother's sleep, would turn the music down in turn.

When we were within twenty minutes of Camp Joslin, I heard rustling from the backseat. Before I had turned around to look at my brother, I knew that he was not just stirring from a restful sleep. I could hear the twitching of my brother's body as his clothes rubbed against the seat's cloth. Sure enough, the music from the car radio was suddenly drowned out with screams from the backseat. This was not good. I was alone with Mom, my brother was screaming and shaking, and we were in a car going sixty-five miles per hour down the Mass Pike.

Mom immediately told me to jump into the backseat with Jon. I did not hesitate. Swinging my body between the front seats, I slid next to my trembling brother in the back. When I got back there, I immediately recognized the signs that this was going to be a very bad reaction.

My brother's eyes were glued shut and his body jerked in sharp, violent motions.

While I was sliding into the backseat, Mom reached across the front seat I had left behind and opened the glove compartment of her car. Here, alongside maps and miscellaneous papers, was a generous supply of those ubiquitous honey packets. While holding the wheel steady with her left hand, she grabbed a fistful of plastic and thrust her right arm between the seats so that I could take the packets. This time, I would be more than the toast maker.

With the honey packets delivered, my mom's arm returned to the wheel and her foot pressed more heavily against the accelerator. Focused on getting Jon straight to medical help, she spoke to me calmly, dividing her attention between looking back at us through her rearview mirror and watching the highway in front of us.

Mom coached me as I pressed my body against my brother's jerking movements and tore open the first honey packet. When Jon's mouth opened with a scream, I thrust the packet into the side of his mouth and squeezed. I could feel the sticky honey ooze through the plastic and into my brother's mouth. His jaw clamped tight and a small gurgle came from somewhere; then it opened again with another scream.

I emptied the honey packets one by one into my brother's mouth and even employed my mom's brave finger technique once or twice. Jon's screams and shaking did not subside despite my efforts. All at once, through slits in my brother's eyes, I saw his eyeballs roll back into his head. He was having a seizure.

Panicked, I told Mom what I had seen, but somehow I think she had sensed it was coming. I could feel the car lurch forward as she again increased the pressure on the accelerator. Her voice still calm, Mom told me to put my arms around my brother and hold him as his body jerked. Then she debated with herself aloud whether she should take the exit for the hospital in Worchester or continue a few more miles to Camp Joslin.

In the end, Camp Joslin won out. Our car sped down the highway, off the exit, and through winding back roads until we finally reached the narrow driveway into the camp. All the while, I held my brother's seizing body in the backseat of the car.

Driving into camp, Mom frantically beeped her horn while she rolled down her window and yelled to the first adult she saw. We drove past the lake and basketball pavilion, past the cabins and the dining hall, onto a narrow dirt drive, and directly to the camp infirmary. Finally, the car stopped, and in a flash Mom was out her door and into the backseat. The camp director was there, along with several nurses, the camp doctor, and a few counselors who had run behind the car as it wound through the camp property. With their help, Jon was lifted out of my arms and into the infirmary.

I left the backseat too and followed the group into the infirmary. I stopped short of heading back to the room where they took Jon. Instead, I stood around in the lobby of the building and listened as the professionals and my mom worked on my brother. As I recall, it took quite a while — something like twenty more minutes — but they brought my brother around without resorting to the dreaded glucagon shot.

When the commotion ended and I saw one of the counselors head to the dining room to get Jon a snack, I left the lobby and went to sit on one of the rocking chairs that adorned the large front porch of the infirmary. Within a few minutes, the counselor came back with the food. I stared out onto the green lawn in front of me. After a little while longer, a few counselors came out with Jon walking among them. They

60

were laughing and ran down the porch stairs and off into the woods to join some camp activity already in progress.

I sat on the porch and watched them leave. I then began to cry. A few minutes later, the camp director came through the infirmary doors and onto the porch. He stopped when he saw me sitting there weeping. Without hesitating, he pulled up a chair next to mine, put his arm on my shoulder, and told me I had done a good job. I continued to sob.

When a person with diabetes has too much insulin and not enough glucose in the blood, an insulin reaction occurs. These can be quite scary, as I have related. If the blood sugar is not low and not just right, it is, naturally, high.

For the observer, the outward signs of high blood sugar are subtler than its opposite. There are no scary episodes of uncontrollable shaking. There are no terrifying screams. There are no seizures. The danger presented by high blood sugar, while infinitely greater than that of low blood sugar, is a quiet one. The body's response to high blood sugar is to shut down. If the high is prolonged or too severe, a diabetic coma sets in and the possibility of death looms.

Therefore, my memories of my brother's battles with high blood sugar are few, though those battles were, unfortunately, not rare. Those episodes were marked with lethargy and sickness. These were horrible times for Jon, but for me they were more welcome than the wrenching reactions. Now, some thirty years beyond those early battles with diabetes, I realize how much peril my brother was in when his blood sugar spiked and stubbornly refused to come down from lofty heights.

Barring some accident brought on by the uncontrollable physical wrenching of the reaction that resulted from low blood sugar, like the always-feared fall or car accident, my brother's body would, as discussed previously, eventually kick in and break down stored fats to raise the blood sugar level to normal. There was no such self-help when it came to the highs. Left untreated, high blood sugar means death. This is why a diagnosis of diabetes one hundred years ago, before the discovery of insulin, was a terminal one.

From a child's and later a self-concerned teenager's perspective, though, high blood sugar was better than low blood sugar. Highs meant I could go about my business. Highs did not wake me up at in the middle of the night. Highs were silent. While my brother and mom had different feelings than I did, highs were fine with me.

Chapter Eight

———∾———

GROUND RULES

From my birth in March 1972 until Jon's diabetes diagnosis in January 1980, my childhood was, to a great degree, normal. Everything changed after that winter day of diagnosis. My brother changed. My parents changed. Our family was never the same.

These, then, were the ground rules of my childhood after January 11, 1980:

- During the daylight hours, when I was with my brother, I was constantly on the lookout for any sign that would indicate his blood sugar was dropping.

- I slept most soundly early in the night.

- After midnight, light sleep was the rule, and I was ever ready to jump out of bed and follow my parents toward the screaming.

- Nighttime reactions meant I would eventually be called upon to make toast in the wee hours of the morning.

- Juice was all but gone from our house, reserved for treatment of Jon's low blood sugar and insulin reactions. Diet soda ruled the day.

- Sugary snacks and desserts were hidden, available only when my brother was asleep or away.

- If my brother appeared when sweets were being enjoyed, sweets were hidden and our enjoyment was suspended.

- Snacks were allowed at almost all times of the day, including before bed, provided they were healthy and sugar-free.

- Traditionally sweet-filled holidays such as Halloween and Easter now meant real presents rather than sugary junk.

- The kitchen and laundry room, once the sole territory of my mom, was now the home of space dedicated to my brother.

- Breakfast and dinner began with the ceremony of blood sugar testing and insulin shots, and what Jon — and often the rest of the family — ate was often based on American Diabetes Association guidelines.

- Glove compartments, purses, and my backpack for school became repositories for honey packets, just in case.

- If a reaction was severe, I cried and shook when it was over. My brother ran out ready to play.

- A large poster with the outline of my brother's body hung on walls or doors to track shots.

- School, summer camp, and my grandmother's house were all escapes.

In addition to these ground rules, other changes were made over time and I felt guided by these unspoken rules:

- There was a hierarchy of feeding; if necessary, my brother's food came first no matter how hungry I or others might be.

- Our growth was no longer measured physically along the basement door and shouldn't be discussed for fear of unsavory comparisons.

- A cold or stomach virus for me was no big deal, although it could be a tool that forced adults to shift their attention. If contracted by Jon, it immediately became a big deal.

- No matter what happened to me, I was to be thankful that I was spared the disease borne by Jon.

- Equality between brothers became that of outcome, not opportunity.

- I was to strive to be perfect, so as to avoid further disruption to a family already burdened with chronic disease.

- Attention was awarded for excelling, being bad, or being sick.

- My most important job was to take care of my brother.

PART TWO
SHADOW CHILD

Chapter Nine

———— ∾∾ ————

RELATIONSHIP CHANGES

The introduction of diabetes and its quick ascendancy to starring role within our family changed more than our habits and processes. In fundamental ways, diabetes altered our relationships with one another.

In January 1980, my mom, my dad, and I were all unaware of the relationship changes that my brother's diagnoses was about to thrust upon us. Within a matter of days, it was easy for my parents to see the structural changes that would be necessary to accommodate our new, unwanted family member. I suspect, though, that they did not foresee the way the disease would soon modify the balance of our family and dictate new rules for its members. As a child of seven going on eight years old, I was not prepared for such changes.

Diabetes not only changed the infrastructure of our family; it also changed the rules. It's as if my family was traveling down one road and suddenly was swooped up and placed on a different road, in a different direction. But diabetes did not stop there. Not only were we placed on an entirely new road, the rules of the new road were different from that of the old, familiar one. Some of these rules contradicted the old ones. Other rules looked familiar but changed subtly on the new road on which we were placed.

While the changes to relationships and rules were less anticipated, their appearance within our family only slightly lagged behind the changes to infrastructure. Within weeks, many of these changes were apparent to even me, the almost-eight-year-old brother. The Mom and Dad I had known before diagnosis day were gone and replaced with post-diagnosis doppelgangers. Our parent–child relationships changed rapidly. Looking back, the changed relationship between my mother and me seems more startling and obvious. Diabetes, though, is thorough, and my relationship with my father was altered as well.

My relationship with my brother Jon changed more gradually. For much of our early adolescence, our relationship remained that of typical brothers. We played, we fought, we played some more. During those early years, the most noticeable change in my relationship with Jon was the increased sense of responsibility and caregiving that manifested itself within me, as it did within every member of our family. While my share of responsibility and care had always been roughly proportionate to my age, it was enhanced considerably following my brother's diagnosis. It was not until I became a teenager, however, that diabetes took its most drastic toll on my relationship with Jon.

As the following chapters explore the impact diabetes had on the relationships between my family members and me, I believe the first sentences of this book bear repeating. There are no bad humans in this story. There are no malignant siblings or abusive parents to be found in the pages that follow. The villain is the chronic disease, and even it acts without malice. This is not a story of blame. This is a story of survival and adaptation.

Chapter Ten

———∞∞———

MOTHER

My memories of my mother before January 11, 1980, are sparse but joyful and content. As the firstborn, I have the comforting feelings of being the apple of my mother's eye and the sole recipient of her parental devotions before my brother's birth. Because I was only three when my brother was born, my assessment of my early relationship with my mother is based primarily on family stories, happy photographs, and the absence of negative feelings.

While I believe it is safe to say that, like most firstborns, the advent of my younger sibling brought some confusion and adjustment, my relationship with my mother continued to be a typical, healthy one after my brother's birth. Even the diagnosis of my two-year-old brother with juvenile rheumatoid arthritis (JRA) and his subsequent treatment did not result in changes between my mother and me that were substantial enough to be burned into memory. JRA brought a leg brace and bottles upon bottles of pink children's aspirin into my young life, but it did not alter my relationship with my mother.

The four years following my brother's birth were happy ones for our family. My mother, like all mothers, faced the challenges of caring for two children, but that was not unexpected. Because she had been an only child, I suspect that it took my mother time to learn the normal play–fight–play rhythms of brothers, but she accomplished that with seeming ease.

Diabetes was not JRA though. Its unwanted entry into our family in the winter of 1980 was not akin to the equally unwelcome introduction of JRA. Diabetes was something entirely different, and the road it placed my mother and me on was as unfamiliar as it was unwelcome.

Diabetes is selfish. The disease that attacked my brother demanded my mother's full attention. This was not a disease that was easily managed. Administering proper insulin dosages was trickier than doling out children's aspirin. Diabetes would never go into remission, as JRA did. Diabetes demanded a full-time mother. Where did that leave me?

In retrospect, I was often left on the sidelines. How could my mother care for my younger, diabetic brother as well as she needed to and did and still devote the same amount of time and resources to me, the healthy, older son? The answer is simply that she could not. No one in her position could. What she did, I believe, was rationally assess the situation that confronted her and the resources available to her. She then distributed those resources between Jon and me as best as she could. I doubt that this was a conscience effort on her part. Rather, like most mothers, she did the best she could for her two boys in the best way that she knew how.

Naturally, a four-year-old boy has slightly different requirements of his mother than does a seven-year-old boy. Add diabetes into that mix, and the distance between those requirements expands exponentially.

Some differences between my needs and those of Jon were obvious.

For example, when it came to food, we both needed to be provided with breakfast, lunch, and dinner and with occasional snacks between meals. But after the diagnosis, the specifics of those needs rapidly diverged. If I went without a snack or if a meal was delayed, I might be upset but I would be okay. If Jon went without a snack or properly timed meal, and if the food did not meet the requirements dictated by his insulin dose, his blood sugar would drop drastically, resulting in too much insulin in his bloodstream and an insulin reaction. Being upset and going into convulsions are two different results from the same act. The solution was simple: When it came to food, my brother was given priority.

The food example seems obvious and perhaps, at first blush, rather innocuous. But put yourself in the shoes of the hungry, eight-year-old boy and then those of his mother. The patience and understanding of a hungry child is, as all parents know, limited. In his eyes, he is hungry and needs to eat — period. If he is made to wait for what he needs until after his younger sibling has been fed, happy times are not in the cards. Tempers and tears are the natural course in those situations. Magnify that occurrence into something less than constant but much more than rare, and a ready-made formula for the creation of jealousy, resentment, and self-doubt becomes fairly obvious.

Placing yourself in the shoes of the mother in our example is no cheerier. No mother wants to deny her child something as basic as food for even a few minutes. As parents, when our children are hungry, we react innately and seek to satisfy their needs. Having to tell your child he has to wait to eat until his younger sibling is fed cannot be easy. Again, imagine having to say those words regularly and then repeatedly deal with the unpleasant aftermath.

While I am sure the food issue left lasting marks on my subconscious, it is not a subject that I often think of when my mind wanders back through those early years. However, the food dilemma has remained fresh in my mother's mind. It was even one of the first stories she told my wife when we began dating. Without solicitation, my mother expressed her concern that "Randall always felt cheated" in those situations and how upsetting that had been for her. These statements were made to my wife-to-be some thirty years after the food dilemmas occurred. Clearly, the uneven distribution diabetes demanded of even the simplest of resources had a lasting impact on my mother.

There were other basic resources that my mother had to ration. As most parents with two or more children will admit, both mothers and fathers tend to devote more vigilant attention to the initial health of their firstborn than their second, third, and so on. I remember well when my firstborn, three-month-old son fell off the bed. That fall resulted in a trip to the emergency room by frantically concerned parents. My son was fine. We were just overprotective and under experienced parents.

Though I don't recall my second son falling off the bed, I am confident that if he had his mother and I would have picked him up, brushed away the tears, and observed him for a reasonable time to make sure he was okay. We had some experience under our belt and understood that kids are tough and in most cases will be fine.

That was most likely the case with my parents, my brother, and me for the first four years of my brother's life, despite the introduction of JRA into our lives during that early period. The advent of diabetes in our family, though, turned that learned experience of my parents on its head. Any hardening experience regarding health issues that my mother had gained through the collective eleven-year existence of my brother and me went out the window. Overnight, Jon became the fragile child – the firstborn that he never was.

My mother's parental vigilance went into overdrive when it came to

Jon. This was a natural reaction to the diagnosis of such a difficult, chronic disease. My brother would be fine as long as he and his diabetes were carefully managed. The task of managing Jon and his diabetes fell almost exclusively to my mother throughout his childhood and teenage years.

Still, no matter how much she might try, my mother only had a given amount of energy and time to devote to the demands of diabetes. One's vigilance can be stretched only so far, and it quickly became another resource that my mother had to ration between her sons. As the healthy, older child, the amount of watchfulness she could spare for me had to be limited. The vast amount of my mother's vigilance had to be directed to my younger, sick brother.

In this way, from my perspective, my baby brother fast became my babied brother in many ways. Jon's well-being became my mother's number one priority, and his happiness became her second. The two, health and happiness, seemed to go hand in hand when it came to my mother's view of Jon. I am confident that my mother wished the same for me then and does to this day. The difference was that she had to be actively engaged in the management of my brother's health and in doing so became actively engaged in the management of his happiness.

This extended motherly attention is something that all children love to receive—and once they have it, they don't want to let it go. It is the rare child who will readily give up being the center of all things.

A new dynamic developed between my mother and my brother within our family. Jon's illness demanded my mother's full attention and management. That need naturally resulted in the devotion of my mother to my brother and his health. From there, it extended into Jon's happiness.

The Saturday mornings of my childhood serve as a terrific example of how this dynamic worked in both positive and negative ways. These mornings arrived early, with all four members of our family typically rising by 6:00 a.m. My brother and I would eat our breakfast, get dressed, and immediately plop ourselves down on the couch to watch the Saturday morning cartoons. When I tell my own children that when I grew up cartoons were on once a week on Saturday morning, they look at me like I must be from the Bronze Age. Nonetheless, those of you born in the 1970s and earlier know that this was the state of affairs of TV animation in the years before the advent of cable television.

My time in front of the television on Saturday morning was always limited because as soon as my father was done with breakfast, he would shower, dress, and be ready to start the day's work. The day's work, no matter what it consisted of, nearly always involved me.

My father would come down stairs, put his work boots on, and ask whether I was ready to go. I say that my father asked, but it was always understood that I had little choice in the matter. It was a given that I would join him in his day's chores and projects. The opposite was true for my younger brother.

Throughout our childhood, I was expected to work alongside my father, while Jon's participation was optional. I say optional, but that is a bit unfair. I am sure that on most of those Saturday mornings my brother truly did not feel well, his blood sugar being either too high or too low. When your blood sugar is out of whack, you don't feel like doing much at all. Additionally, I suspect that there were two other forces at play when it came to Jon's optional participation – my father's sense of fear and desire for convenience.

My mother made the ultimate determination of whether Jon would join my father and me or remain at home. This decision was weighed heavily with input from my brother. Cartoons or chores? Not always a tough decision for a young boy to make.

Still, my mother was always ready to defend his choice. In my young eyes, she stood at the decision-making gate and handed my brother free passes that were never made available to me. It just was not fair.

~~~

When faced with a perceived injustice, humans, including young children, generally find clever ways to overcoming that state of inequity. And so, as a child, I set out to find ways in which I could even the playing field and gain more of my mother's attention, if not devotion, than I had been rationed. To my young mind, the formula became simple: Illness equaled attention, while health negated it. To win more attention from my mother, then, I needed to be sick.

Seeking a more equal footing with my younger brother on the maternal attention scale led to many instances of feigned illnesses. None of these faux maladies were serious; I was not daring enough to attempt that much acting. Still, they were enough to take me out of school, keep me home from school, or allow me to stay on the couch watching cartoons on Saturday mornings. It was not school or work that I was trying to escape during these episodes. I was not trying to escape anything. I was trying to gain back some of the attention that I believed diabetes had stolen from me.

In elementary school, I became a regular visitor to the nurse's office. Usually the reason for my visit was a stomach malady. It seemed my stomach was upset a lot during those early days. The drill was always the same in the small room tucked in a corner of the elementary school next to the principal's office. I would walk in looking as sick to my stomach as I could muster and register my complaint. The nurse would look me over; invite me to lay down on the small, screened cot behind her desk; and take my temperature. My temperature was always an issue. I remember few visits to that office when the thermometer actually rose above normal. Had it been a rectal thermometer, I am confident that the frequency of my trips to the nurse's office would have been drastically reduced.

After the thermometer inevitably failed to help my case, the nurse would usually have me sit or lie down for a while to see whether I felt better with a bit of time. After that, I had a fifty-fifty shot at being sent home. When I was sent not home but back to class, I slowly moped out of the nurse's office and back through the halls to my classroom. While the ultimate goal of going home had not been achieved, I still had gained attention from the school nurse for twenty or thirty minutes. That was better than nothing.

A little less than half of my visits to the school nurse were successful. By successful, I mean that those visits resulted in a call to my mother or father explaining the situation and asking them to pick me up early from school. Most of the time, it was my mother, grandmother, or great-aunt who drove to school and picked me up. My mother was often teaching and, when my grandmother or great-aunt was unavailable, had to either leave her class early or find a substitute. Either way, my illness meant that someone would have to drive me home—a good twenty-mile trip from school—and then drive another twenty miles to pick up my brother from the same school upon normal dismissal.

My need to get home and receive some attention was costly in time, productivity, and gas for the adults in my life. In retrospect, I can appreciate the costs of my behavior now. As an elementary school kid, those costs did not cross my mind. I was looking for more maternal attention, and I knew that being sick was the one way I would get some.

Did my mother, father, grandmother, or great-aunt, or the school nurse, understand what was going on? I am sure that to some extent they did. My visits to the school nurse were frequent enough to win me a trip to the allergist to test for various food allergies. I was subjected to numerous pin pricks in my arms and tested positive for tomatoes.

When I was thirteen, I hit the attention jackpot. I really did have a stomachache that time. The trip to the same nurse's office resulted in a positive temperature reading and a pretty quick trip to the hospital in Burlington. Though in pain, imagine how pleased I was to be a patient at the same place my brother visited regularly.

At the hospital, after several x-rays and three rectal exams by three different doctors (and thus three different sets of fingers), it was determined that I had appendicitis and required surgery. That ordeal got me a hospital stay and a week home from school. My mother stayed with me in the hospital and for much of the week I was at home. It was awesome with respect to the time and care my mother gave me but not so awesome with respect to the rest. It really did hurt.

Years after my appendix decided it needed to flame up, there is sometimes a lingering question in the back of my mind of whether this was a typical "stomachache" gone awry. But, after consideration, I always dismiss that possibility outright. Even if all of the medial personnel decided to turn a blind eye to my feint and do some unnecessary surgery, there were still the three rectal exams. Had I been faking, the first set of fingers would have been enough. The gig would have been up before the second and third sets got near their target.

I don't recall further "stomach illnesses" that brought me to the nurse's office following my appendectomy. Soon after, I was a teenager, and my needs for greater maternal attention — or at least my mechanisms for obtaining such attention — changed. I also had a lot more to do in school that I did not want to miss out on, sports and girlfriends being two of the most prominent. As a teenager, I realized there was another surefire formula when it came to gaining attention from my mother, albeit negative attention.

∿

My mother was and remains a person of abundant resources and energy. I was not abandoned and left to fend for myself when it came to my adolescent and teenage life. While diabetes demanded much of her time, care, and compassion, she still had her eye on me. Excellence and enforcement were among the drives my mother directed at me. I still fell under her watchful eye when it came to doing well in school and behaving in an approved and appropriate manner.

As early as elementary school, my mother made it clear that my focus was to be on excelling in elementary school, high school, college, and graduate school. That was my job while I lived under her roof and through her finances. To her credit, my mother did not assign this task and then turn her back and expect miracles. In these matters, she was constantly attentive and determined to see me through.

My mother was incredibly supportive of my academic efforts throughout those years. If I needed help with school at any stage, she either helped me herself or found someone with the skill set to do so. When I got home from school or sports practice, my first task was to complete my homework. My mother's task was to make sure I did so. When I faced my first college papers, my mother left my brother at home with my father, drove two-and-a-half hours, and stayed the night in a hotel room near campus to make sure that I had completed my papers to the best of my ability.

Like academic performance, when it came to discipline, I was never far from my mother's watchful eye. This was only an extension of her mantra of academic excellence. My mother wanted nothing to prevent me from excelling first in school and later in life. Bad behavior was not tolerated.

I was to be a polite boy and then young man. My hair was never to be too long. Piercings (at that time limited to boys' ears), and ripped jeans were not tolerated. There was a dress code to be followed under my parents, and failure to follow it was not an option. The reason that my mother always gave for these rules, if I asked, was that society would be looking at me and that I wanted them to see me at my best at all times. Businessmen did not have earrings or long hair. Ripped jeans were not acceptable in the office and so were not acceptable in my teenage wardrobe.

Those were the little things that my mother attended to. Big disciplinarian issues were not even conceivable. Teenage drinking was not tolerated. Teenage sex was not tolerated. Any activity that was illegal (drugs, crime, etc.) was not tolerated. My mother made it clear to me that the consequences for any of these ill-fated actions would be severe. Severe ranged from no support and no college to being kicked out of the house. From elementary school and through graduation from college, I firmly believed that my parents would follow through with these declared consequences.

The emphasis on academic excellence to prepare me for a career, the all-encompassing discipline and enforcement shroud that my mother hung over me, and even her strong-willed support led to the development of a businesslike relationship between my mother and me. In effect, my mother became my first boss. As her son, my job was to perform to the best of my abilities in school and to produce high grades. I was rewarded with attention and praise when I achieved my goals. If I failed to reach my goals, the rewards were not there. If I allowed myself to go awry and break the rules, disciplinary actions would be taken, including the possibility of being fired.

As a teenager, this businesslike relationship with my mother led me to the realization that if I simply did enough to appease her, I would be largely left alone, the desire of any teen with a watchful parent. The goal then became to make my mother happy so that I could do what I wanted to do. Whether her happiness came from my excelling academically or from my feigned personal purity and perfection, all I began to care about when it came to my mother was whether she was pleased with me. If she was pleased, I was free. If she was unhappy, my world would not be good until she was happy with me again.

This relationship with my mother had its benefits. With her support and drive, I excelled academically and otherwise throughout elementary school and high school. This led to acceptance to great colleges, with attendance at a good liberal arts college followed by a top twenty-five law school. Her focus on discipline and my belief in the stated consequences of failure kept me pretty damn clean throughout my teenage years and college. Apart from keeping me out of the petty crimes, drinking, and drugs that too often plague young adults, under my mother's influence I was a clean-cut, polite, and well-mannered young man.

At times, though, it seems that my relationship with my mother lacked a degree of comfort, compassion, and doting. As a young child and teenager, I often felt that my mother directed those resources nearly exclusively to my brother. Her need to care for Jon and manage his diabetes when, because of his age, he could not do so, drained her. She did not abandon me, but she could share with me only those resources that she had left after so much of her energies were absorbed by my younger brother and his diabetes.

Ultimately, I have done well in school and life. I have a strong career and am, by all accounts, a successful, forty-four-year-old adult. The resources that my mother devoted to me, and that helped me get where

I am, however, are no longer needed. With her help, I have successfully developed my own well-honed drive and discipline.

This begs the question, what remains of my relationship with my mother when it is based on elements that are now to a large extent expired? The answer to that question is that without some serious re-working and relearning, our relationship today would have little substance. Beyond the basis of love that always exists between mother and son, as well as the great deal of respect and gratitude that I have for my mother, much of the foundation of our early relationship aged out.

Growing older – and in many respects, wiser — I realized in my young adulthood that many of my earlier perceptions of my relationship with my mother were false. The demands of chronic disease had tainted my vision. My mother is an exceptional person and an amazing parent. The loss of love and devotion that I had once perceived never occurred in reality, though diabetes placed much of it in the shadows.

Chapter Eleven

FATHER

Though at the time I would have done just about anything to stay on the couch and watch cartoons with my brother Jon all of those Saturday mornings, by being forced out of the house I was forced into a different relationship with my father. In hind sight, I am glad that I was made to join my father all of those weekends. I learned so much from working alongside of him. That knowledge is continually put to work now that my wife and I own a large, old house in constant need of attention.

This relationship with my father began earlier than my brother's birth and diagnosis with diabetes. Looking back through the old family albums reveals many Kodak moments of me "helping" my father with the restoration of either our old farmhouse or furniture in my father's workshop. Each of those photos shows a happy two- or three-year-old and, usually in the background, a happy young dad.

When diabetes struck our family, it brought me closer to my father even as it intruded on my relationship with my mother. I was with my father the day my mother and Jon heard the diagnosis of diabetes. I was with my father the initial week that Jon and my mother spent in the Burlington hospital learning how to cope with the disease. I was with my father many of the days and nights that Jon and my mother spent in Burlington either in the hospital or attending doctors' appointments.

I believe my father tried to avoid diabetes as much as he could. He never learned to give Jon shots by himself, and only took on that daily duty when directed and assisted by my mother. My father did learn to handle Jon's insulin reactions both solo and as an assistant to my mother. Though at one time a pretty hard sleeper, my father always sprang from his bed and either led or closely followed my mother for the short trip down the hall to my brother's room.

Despite his adoption of the changes my brother's diabetes brought to our family, my father was and remains a child of the 1940s and a conservative man of the 1960s and 1970s. He was not a touchy-feely man. I don't think he ever changed our diapers, and I know pancakes formed the one meal he could successfully cook by himself. When it came to housekeeping, he did no better. I distinctly remember him cleaning up a mess on our family room carpet with bleach.

Because my father is not a big sports fan, there were no Saturday night baseball or Sunday afternoon football games to watch. He rarely drank and did not smoke. Instead, my father's love is to be out of the house—working on his property, tinkering with his antique cars, or refinishing or making furniture in his workshop. If you wanted to spend time with my father, you needed to be out of the house working with him. Otherwise, you could try to catch a few words with him early in the morning or in the evening.

This presented a challenge for my young brother. There was rarely a reason I should not go somewhere or do something with my father, so that is what I did. In contrast, Jon was more likely to be found in or around the house because he did not feel well. Diabetes deprived my brother of much of the early work experiences and adventures that I shared with my father.

As I mentioned previously, I believe that my father's own fears and desire for convenience also separated him from my brother. Bringing Jon along to work in the woods, for instance, meant the possibility of having to deal with a scary insulin reaction. It definitely meant having to be more diligent about snacks and meal times. I have the feeling my father avoided these things as much as possible.

Our relationships with our parents became mirror images of one another. Diabetes brought Jon and my mother closer and formed strong bonds between them. Diabetes brought my father and me closer and formed a strong work bond between the two of us. These were not conscience decisions on any of our parts. These disparate relationships formed as a direct result of diabetes' influence on our family.

Nor were these temporary or trivial developments. For many years, when the four of us were together, it was clear that diabetes had a permanent impact on our family structure. When we gathered, my mother and brother were almost always hovering near each other, while my father and I did the same. The separation into these mother–son and father–son pairs was unusual and prevalent enough that it did not go unnoticed. New acquaintances to this dynamic often made some questioning remark—indirect or direct. Some of these remarks initially led me to evaluate the impact diabetes had on our family on a deeper level.

Chapter Twelve

Brother: The First Six Years

The introduction of diabetes into our family has had the greatest impact on my relationship with the target of the disease, my brother Jon. Diabetes swept our relationship into currents that I am positive would not have flowed through our family but for that wretched disease.

The disease took my brother and me through several distinct phases as we grew up together, each with its own twists and complications. The first was our relationship when we were both very young, and the second phase began during my years in high school and continued until my mid-thirties. Throughout these two phases, diabetes was the unwanted third person in our relationship. Diabetes truly proved the axiom that two's company but three's a crowd. It also shaped the third phase, where Jon and I find ourselves today.

After Jon's diagnosis, my relationship initially remained fairly typical.

The play–fight–play rhythm that we had fallen into before the diagnosis continued. When Jon was old enough, he and I attended the same elementary school, and after school we would spend our time playing in the woods until dinner in the winter and until dusk in the spring and fall. In the summer, unless it rained, we spent hours upon hours playing outside or swimming in our pond.

Lest you think I paint an idyllic picture, let me assure you that Jon and I had some ferocious, drag-out fights during those summer days and after-school afternoons. In fact, I am sure that we averaged one or two a day. These were normal battles between brothers. There needn't be a rational cause for the arguments, as all parents come to understand. They just tend to happen.

No matter how fierce a fight might have been, to our credit my brother and I did not spend much time being mad afterward. I have many vivid memories of slamming the door to my room, or my brother slamming his, pledging our hate for each other aloud and swearing never to play or talk to the other again. All of our angry pledges fell flat within ten or twenty minutes. Whoever had been the aggressor would usually open his door, approach the sibling's room, and slip a note under the door.

Those notes most often simply said "I am sorry, let's play" in our elementary school scrawl. Occasionally, such notes were greeted with some huffing and puffing from the other side of the door and it took additional verbal assuaging or perhaps another, sweeter note to bring the other brother around. Within a half hour of the fight, though, Jon and I were back to being best friends and resuming whatever activity we were engaged in before one of us decided that he hated the other.

That, in a nutshell, was our young relationship cycle before diabetes and for a couple of years following the diagnosis. On the whole, my brother and I were happy in each other's company. Our physical distance from our school friends and even nearest neighbor tended to prevent Jon and me from engaging in long-term grudge matches. It was either play with each other or play alone. Most of the time, playing alone was not fun after the first ten minutes or so. When we were at home, Jon and I were together.

～～

Unless it was raining or bitterly cold, we were together outdoors. Jon and I had many, many forts established in the woods surrounding our house. The two most notable of these were The Rock and Jon's Camp. The Rock was just that, a large rock located in the middle of an old stone wall that was overgrown with small trees and brush. The site was only about two hundred feet from the back of our house. If our mother peered through the brush and branches, she could see her two sons playing on The Rock from her kitchen window.

Jon and I spent hours playing at The Rock. We played war games and other games known only to young, country boys. Sometimes, during the summer, my mother would pack us a lunch that we would take out to the Rock for a picnic. The Rock was as simple as it gets, and it brought us a great deal of joy.

Jon's Camp was a bit of a step up. It was located just inside the wood's edge in the rear of our property. We could not see the house from the site, and my mother could not see us. Compared to The Rock, the siting of Jon's Camp was a declaration of independence for Jon and me.

The camp was also a bit more involved than a large rock in a stone wall. Jon and I cleared a small section of territory just inside the woods, about fifteen feet from the edge of the back lawn. After we had the area cleared, we hauled flat stones from the nearby brook and built a primitive fire pit. With the help of our great-aunt Alfreda, we used dead branches and old boards from a long-expired farm dump to create a lean-to shelter that completed the site. This was Jon's Camp. Once up and running, it was the site of many hours of play for us. My mother packed our lunches for Jon's Camp, just as she had for The Rock.

Beyond The Rock and Jon's Camp, our other focus during the summer months was the pond. The pond was one of two on our property and consisted of about an acre of fresh water supplied by the brook that ran past Jon's Camp. The pond was located a mere fifty feet or so from our house and spread out toward the rear of the property and Jon's Camp. Just following my brother's diagnosis, my parents had the pond drained and dredged, making it clean and swimmable.

In addition to deepening the water, my parents brought in a few dump truck loads of sand, creating a more pleasant bottom and a beach area from which my brother and I based our aquatic fun. Add in a perpetually growing fleet of rubber rafts, and a floating wooden platform with ladder for diving or jumping into the deepest part of the pond, and we had a recipe for unending summer fun. Some days we were in the pond from midmorning until the evening, nonstop. We often ate our lunches on the beach or even the large, rounded boulder that protruded from the middle of the pond.

As we grew older and more independent in our play, however, I felt increasingly responsible for and protective of Jon. At the age of eight or nine, I became something more than a sibling but less than a parent. I saw myself as the older, healthy brother and Jon as the younger brother who had serious health issues. Jon's health problems were scary to me, and I knew that if I was not responsible enough, not protective enough, they would raise an ugly head and not only scare the hell out of me but also hurt Jon. As my mother taught me about diabetes and the effects it had on Jon, I became the youngest member of my brother's diabetes management team.

In addition to making toast and helping with insulin reactions, my management role primarily involved an increased vigilance when it came to my brother's mood and behavior, both possible signs of up- or downswings in blood sugar. As his playmate, I was often nearest in proximity to Jon, and I served as a sort of early warning system for my parents. If I remained aware, I might be the first to see telltale signs of a blood sugar swing and alert my parents to the need to take action. That was the plan, anyway.

In practice, my initial success with the early warning role was only about 50 percent. I was very young, and some of the earliest behavioral signs were beyond my detection. I was also usually quite absorbed with whatever game Jon and I were playing. In time, my success rate improved as the bellwethers of blood sugar shifts, particularly low blood sugar, became more familiar to me.

Some of the methods I used to remain vigilant belied both my youth and my status as big brother. One method that stands out in my mind —and, I am confident, my brother's memories — was the punch test for low blood sugar. It was a simple test. I would deliver an out of the blue, fairly hard punch to my brother, usually to the upper arm. The reaction that this elicited from Jon would then give me a good idea of whether his blood sugar was low or on its way there.

As you can imagine, this blood sugar test was not popular with my little brother. I suppose that in its best light, this test was based on the theory that, as the older brother, I was familiar with the correlation between punch weight and verbal reaction. If a certain punch resulted in more verbal outcry than normal, that indicated a low blood sugar. In reality, my rationale for the test was not so scientific. I just liked giving my brother the occasional punch to the shoulder.

The other primary requirement of my role as the youngest member of the diabetes management team was to carry packets of honey or other sugary substances with me every time Jon and I played outdoors. This might seem innocuous, but it wasn't. For one thing, a young boy only has so many pockets, and those pockets are in high demand. I needed them for stones, sticks, the occasional small creature, and other fun stuff. Having to dedicate a pocket to honey packets was an imposition.

If that wasn't bad enough, rolling around on the ground and other common activities in the woods can cause plastic seals to burst, leaving the carrier with a pocket full of sticky honey. This unhappy circumstance was probably hardest on my mother, who had the task of washing the honey out of the pocket. It is never pleasant though when, forgetting about the burst packet, you stick your hand in a pocket and withdraw sticky, honey-covered fingers.

I make light of these tasks now, but they were important back then and forced an increased sense of responsibility onto me as a young child. I knew I was part of the team. I knew that my brother had needs that went beyond those that naturally resulted from his status as younger sibling. None of this was a crushing load to bear, but it was more than a typical older brother is burdened with. To a greater degree, Jon depended on me and my parents depended on me. I was responsible, and I knew that well.

In opposition to increased responsibility and protectiveness toward Jon, the special status that diabetes seem to thrust upon my younger brother brought increased envy and jealousy into our relationship.

To some degree, jealousy is normal when an only child becomes an older sibling upon the arrival of a new younger brother or sister. These feelings usually disappear as the older child learns that Mom and Dad have enough love to go around. This happened between Jon and me. By the time Jon was four years old and I was seven, I was comfortable that my parents loved us both and that my special station in their lives was preserved.

The diabetes diagnosis in 1980 turned that upside down. Yes, at seven years old and going on eight, I understood that I was the lucky one who had been spared from diabetes. I immediately understood that my brother's diagnosis was not a good thing. As time passed and my family adapted to a new way of life centered on the disease, I learned how difficult the disease made my little brother's life and how scary it could be. I knew all of that. Yet I was still jealous.

The sudden shift in my mother's focus from the two of us to almost entirely Jon and diabetes was an extremely difficult one to swallow. I could not overcome the strong feeling of continually being jilted when it came to her attention.

Many day-to-day events evidenced Jon's special status within our family, often at my expense. Two that remain incredibly vivid involved Jon's Camp and a dog named Cassie.

Jon's Camp, the crude lean-to and fire pit just inside the woods at the back of our property, had long been a dedicated base of operations for our play. But over time, Jon showed a growing interest in camps and log cabins that he saw in books, on television, and at Camp Joslin, the diabetes camp he attended for weeks in summers. At some point, my parents made the decision to build a log playhouse that could replace our cobbled-together lean-to.

When I tell you that a real log cabin was built for my brother, I am not exaggerating. The process began with a substantial widening of the clearing that Jon and I had made. Trees were cut, and brush was removed. A concrete slab floor was poured at the site. After it had cured, cedar logs were brought from a property a mile or so down the road that my father had purchased for resale. The logs were cut and hewn to measure, and the construction of the exterior walls begun. Four working, glass windows and a solid door were included in the two-story structure. The installation of an asphalt-shingle, steeply pitched roof was the final step in the construction of the new building.

When all was said and done, my brother's interest in log cabins resulted in the construction of a very nice log playhouse. A couch, table, and cupboard were placed on the first floor of the small building, and two mattresses were carried up to the second. The makeshift stone fire pit that my brother and I had thrown together was replaced with a substantial stone structure that resembled those found in public campgrounds. A picnic table was supplied for the outside of the cabin to accommodate the many lunches and snacks that would be eaten at the site. The site was redubbed Jon's Cabin and has borne that name ever since.

While the site that Jon and I had cleared and built the feeble lean-to fort was always called Jon's Camp, it had been shared between us. Though humble, it was the result of our joint efforts. Jon's Cabin was different. While I remember working on the project, its genesis and construction were adult based, and it was built to respond to my brother's fancy. Unlike Jon's Camp, I had no real sense of ownership when it came to Jon's Cabin. The cabin was built for Jon, not me. It was his alone.

I don't remember ever voicing opposition to the creation of Jon's Cabin. Jon and I continued to play in and around the building, but it was different. Because it was built for him, Jon was keenly aware that when it came to the cabin he made the decisions. The attribution of ownership was implicit in good times and explicit when things went wrong between the two of us. I was there by invite and permission, not because of any sense of shared accomplishment and ownership.

The log playhouse stands on the same site today and is still faithfully called Jon's Cabin. In fact, my brother's recent marriage featured photographs of the wedding party in front of his cabin, something his new wife had wanted because the cabin meant so much to Jon.

Whenever I have been asked about the small cabin in the woods and why it was not called Jon and Randall's Cabin or just The Cabin, I have faithfully and unquestioningly toed the family line. Jon asked for a cabin and he got one. It was built for my brother. When he did not let me use it, I resorted to my own lean-to fort made from dead trees and brush in the woods nearby.

The dog Cassie is the subject of another vivid memory of my childhood jealousy and envy of my brother. Cassie was a purebred, soft-coated wheaten terrier who came into our family when my brother learned to give himself insulin shots.

The self-administration of insulin shots was, before the advent of the insulin pump that many people with type 1 diabetes use today, a critical step in the path toward self-management in a young diabetic's life. It was a huge step. My brother, at the age of five, could take a syringe, fill it full of the proper amount of two types of insulin, and plunge the sharp needle into his body. Most children that age still cry when forced to endure the occasional needle at the doctor's office. The discipline that my brother had obtained at that age impresses me more and more as time goes on.

As a reward for learning to give himself insulin shots, my brother received Cassie. Cassie arrived as a fluffy, cute puppy, and she lived with us some fifteen years. In time, Cassie became more of my mother's dog then Jon's. Initially, though, like Jon's Cabin, Cassie belonged to Jon.

We had another dog too, a black lab mix named Blackie. Blackie was a drop-off. Her original owner did not want her, so the owner took her for a car ride in the country and dumped her off on the side of the road. I remember well the day Blackie arrived on our lawn and how she playfully chased me around the yard while we waited for my father to come home from work and decide whether we could keep her.

The decision was that Blackie could stay. Though she was never referred to as my dog, Blackie was the closest I ever came to having ownership over a pet as a child.

Thus, when Cassie came to us with the label "Jon's dog," my young ire was raised. Again, Jon had received a special status in our family that I had no access to. Yes, the accomplishment of learning to administer his insulin shots was huge. Yes, my brother deserved to be rewarded. But these were all things that were largely beyond my capacity for rational thinking at that age. To me, in receiving a dog, Jon got another thing that I had never been offered.

In addition to increased responsibility and envy, diabetes introduced the element of fear into our brotherly relationship. I became afraid for and of my brother after the diagnosis. I was afraid that I might lose him.

Though my parents kept most of their fear about diabetes to themselves, I was an alert kid and picked up on some of the implications of the danger the disease had brought into our lives. Diabetes was no laughing matter, and the amount of self-education that my parents went through, as well as their stark seriousness about my brother's condition, brought this home to me.

The insulin reaction was an expression of that danger that I understood well. The screams and bodily thrashing coming from my brother drove home that diabetes was a serious threat to my brother's health and safety. No matter how many times my mother explained to me that, if all else failed, Jon's body would eventually kick in and bring itself out of the reaction, I always saw my parents burst into an all-out sprint to Jon when an insulin reaction began. I could not stop believing that Jon was in danger.

The monthly trips to Burlington for doctor appointments were also indications to me that diabetes was a serious threat to my brother's life. I was young, but I knew Plattsburgh had a hospital and many doctors. Only serious health conditions would be cause for a 140-mile roundtrip that crossed Lake Champlain to a bigger city, with better hospitals and doctors.

It did not take our family long to learn that commonplace health issues, such as a cold or stomach bug, could not be treated as trivial when it came to Jon. Colds and viruses became disruptions in Jon's life and diabetes management that had to be closely monitored. A diabetic kid who can't hold anything down because he caught a bug going around school has more problems than just an upset stomach. Blood sugar has to be monitored more frequently, insulin must be adjusted, and the necessary nutrients have to be administered, sometimes intravenously.

Even cuts and bruises meant more to Jon than to me. Diabetes slowed his young body's ability to heal itself. The bruises Jon got from rough-housing or falling while we skated on the pond in the winter took longer to heal than the bruises I obtained from such activities. Cuts on Jon's skin did not scab over as quickly as mine, leaving him more susceptible to infections. I learned all of this along with the rest of my family.

I became privy to bigger, long-term consequences simply by listening to my parents and other adults talk about diabetes. Blindness was rabid among older people with diabetes. Many diabetics lost arms and legs because of poor circulation that resulted from mismanagement of the disease. Kidney failure was also common. These were serious and scary things! In addition, the life expectancy of people with diabetes was significantly lower than that of healthy people. I can remember lying in my bed late at night, crying over that fact on more than one occasion.

All of this drove home the fact that my brother was in danger as a diabetic. He had to learn to manage his diabetes or the consequences would be severe. We had to help Jon manage his diabetes successfully. I was a part of that "we" and I had to help my brother. It was all scary to me.

The more selfish part of the fear that diabetes brought into my preteen life was a mundane, day-to-day fear of Jon himself. I dreaded any time that my young brother would sleep during the day. It seemed that so many of those naps ended in him screaming and shaking, needing urgent doses of honey or other forms of sugar. I was afraid of the screams and the tremors. They scared me to death.

I also dreaded time alone with my brother when my parents were not nearby, including at my grandmother's house. My grandmother and great-aunt were pretty good at handling Jon's reactions —they started learning as soon as my parents and I did — but they were not as adept as my parents. Other adults, such as the occasional babysitter, were clueless.

All of those instances meant that I had to be more responsive to the insulin reactions. I had to play a role that my mother or my father would usually play and could not be relegated to making toast. These were leading roles that I shunned. I wanted my parents there to handle the big tasks. I wanted to skip out and make some toast, closing the door to the loudest of the screams and scariest of the convulsions.

For my own sake, then, I was afraid of being alone with Jon. If Jon and I spent the night at my grandmother's house, I did not sleep well. If Jon and I spent the night at Jon's Cabin, I did not sleep well, even though my parents were only two hundred yards away. If a babysitter came to our house to allow my parents to have a rare night out, I did not sleep until my parents were home.

Still, I faced those scary situations. I never refused to stay the night at my grandmother's house with Jon. I always said yes when Jon would ask whether I would spend the night with him at his cabin, my presence being a prerequisite for him doing so.

From age seven to thirteen, these elements of responsibility, envy, and fear were ever present when it came to my relationship with Jon. I never stopped being afraid, but I allowed the responsibility I felt and all of the positive things Jon and I shared to allow me to see the scary times through. Despite these heavy weights on our shoulders, we remained close during this time and had a lot of fun together.

Two trophies reveal another dynamic that imbedded itself within our small family of four. As I have discussed elsewhere, the summers of my youth were generally spent outdoors with my brother and at summer camp. For me, summer camps revolved around sports. For many years, I fancied myself a basketball player and attended several day and overnight basketball camps. Later, the favored sport became soccer.

Summer camp for Jon meant Camp Joslin, which I have previously described in detail. I cannot say enough about Camp Joslin and the good it did for my brother and the other boys who were lucky enough to spend a few weeks there each summer. While I spent a week or two focused on one sport, Jon and his campmates got to experience many sports and activities throughout their camp days.

The story of two trophies harks back to one of those warm, childhood summers when I attended basketball camp at Norwich University in Vermont and my brother spent two weeks at Camp Joslin in Massachusetts. My parents wisely scheduled the two camps so that they occurred simultaneously, giving themselves a much needed break from the continual demands of their two boys. The simultaneous end dates of the two camps also allowed my parents to combine trips and pick up Jon and me on the same, busy day.

That particular camp stay proved to be a great one for me. I was assigned to a basketball team with other kids my age and a young man who had coached my team the year before at the same camp. Our team gelled immediately, and with some hard work throughout the week, we won our age division at the camp. Each of the players on that summer team received a beautiful plastic gold trophy adorned with basketball player on top and the words "division champions" across the bottom. It was a triumphant end to a great week of camp.

When my parents arrived to pick me up from Norwich University, my brother was in the car excitedly waiting to see me and share camp stories. The three of them had left Camp Joslin early the same morning and drove north through Massachusetts and Vermont to pick me up. I was excited to see my parents and my brother, show them my shiny trophy, and tell them all about our championship series.

After my father parked the car and spotted me in the crowd of campers waiting for their rides home, Jon got out of the car with my parents and walked toward me. I was walking in their direction, lugging my suitcase in one hand and holding my gold championship trophy in the other. When the four of us met, there were the customary excited greetings, handshakes, and hugs.

My father took my suitcase off of my hands, and the four of us began to walk to our car. I was so excited to show Jon and my parents my trophy that I lifted it up and began to tell them the story of our championship. As I began my story, Jon interrupted by holding up, with equal pride, a trophy of his own. Jon's trophy was of the silver, plastic cup variety, without personalized markings. He proudly blurted out that he had won the trophy playing floor hockey at camp.

The thing was, my little brother was so darn proud of his little prize. He was as happy as I was with my own larger, shinier trophy. I also knew that Jon's camp was all about learning how to live and be successful with diabetes, while mine was simply about basketball.

After hearing about my brother's floor hockey success and seeing his little silver cup, my own excitement regarding my achievement at camp began to quickly fade. The bigger gold trophy that I had been wielding with pride receded against my right hip. I remember wishing I could make it disappear, or at least shrink it considerably.

By the time we made it to car, my father had opened the trunk and was placing my suitcase down next to my brother's footlocker. Before he could shut the lid of the trunk, my hand thrust out and buried my championship trophy under my suitcase. I was not going to bring it with me into the backseat for the ride home. My brother had his trophy there, and we would talk about that.

No one told me to stow my trophy away in the trunk that day. My parents did not tell me to listen to my brother's stories of triumph rather than boast of mine. The specter of diabetes had already seeped into my psyche and silently taken care of all of that. I knew in my heart that I needed to let Jon shine. I needed to celebrate his achievement more than mine. After all, I was the healthy brother. I was the lucky one.

At the end of my year in eighth grade, and Jon's year in fifth grade, we were first and foremost brothers. Diabetes had affected both of our lives and our relationship, but it had not overcome us. We were, by and large, happy with each other and in each other's company. Neither of us knew then that when I entered high school and became a bona fide teenager, our relationship was headed for serious changes.

Chapter Thirteen

BROTHER:
HIGH SCHOOL AND COLLEGE

After eighth grade ended, I was ready for high school and anxious for the next four years to begin. Entering the high school years brings so much change to young men and women, it is often difficult to look back and face who we were before we became freshmen and what we became after.

My high school years can be summarized in three words: academics, sports, and girls. My mother, in her excel mode, had spent much of my year in eighth grade and the following summer weeks driving home that the next four years of high school were critical to the ultimate goal of college success. She actively monitored and guided homework, grades, and extracurricular activities that would help me get into the college of my choice.

My mother's efforts of enforcement also increased. She was determined to eradicate distractions from the goal of academic excellence. My participation in school sports was a privilege. If I could not keep my grades to a satisfactory level, meaning A's, sports were not going to happen for me. If she could have suspended my hormone levels and interest in girls during my high school years, my mother would have. Girls were just another distraction that had the potential to jeopardize my academic achievements.

Fortunately, I maintained good grades throughout high school while playing the sports I loved. Girls made it into the picture too. There were some bumpy roads when it came to some classes that I did not like and some girls that I liked too much, but overall high school was a great time for me.

High school, however, was not so great when it came to my relationship with my brother. As they do for most siblings, the days of playing together in the woods or inside with models and figurines ended as I developed interests Jon could not understand while he remained in the world of grade school adolescence. Unfortunately, our respective interests were not the only thing that changed after I entered high school. Diabetes did not allow our relationship to ride the waves of time naturally. The combination of high school and chronic disease put us on a road that most siblings do not travel.

To understand what I mean by this, it is necessary to revisit some of the tenants of our lives back then. Despite having sophisticated parents, Jon and I grew up as country boys. We were not worldly. This was a time without the Internet and the immediate access to the entire world, both beautiful and ugly, that e-connectivity allows our children today. While we both had friends in and out of school, our lives mainly consisted of going to school and coming home to play together.

It seems silly to refer to this as a simpler time, but in many respects it was. Our lives revolved around each other and our family. Except on evenings when my father's participation on any number of charitable boards prevented his early arrival, all four of us routinely ate dinner together. Our conversations around the dinner table focused on tales from our school days and our parents' workdays. After that, we discussed our plans for the next day or the weekend, followed by politics if there was still food left on anyone's plate.

As for vices, our immediate family was conservative. My father did not smoke and limited himself to one drink on Saturday nights. Though I have some foggy memories of whiskey sours and daiquiris (this was the seventies and early eighties after all) among my mother and her friends, I have no clear memories of my mother drinking and I know she never smoked.

The other regular participants in our family life were my grandmother and my great-aunt, Alfreda. These two, dear women were as straight laced as they came and good Catholics. They joined the family dinner every Saturday and Sunday night, without fail, and their influence on all of our lives cannot be overstated.

The only other window into the world that Jon and I had at that time was television. Still, our television time was limited, and our bedtimes were fairly early. Television for us meant Saturday morning cartoons and, if we were lucky, some kid-friendly programs in the evening. We were both in bed before anything racy came on, and let's face it: television was less racy back then.

So, it's fair to say that Jon and I were pretty innocent growing up. We had little exposure to drinking and none to sex. We knew those things existed, but they were squarely negative. People like us did not drink or do drugs. They did not engage in sex unless they were married. Hell, they didn't even wear tattered jeans or waste precious time on nonproductive activities, as might be arbitrarily defined through tales at the dinner table.

High school changed all of that for me. Even though the class composition had remained almost unchanged since first grade and we did not even shift buildings in our small parochial school, things changed nonetheless. Like most kids, our conversations at school advanced well beyond what had piqued our interest in elementary and middle school. Girls began to dominate locker room talk. Drinking and drugs were talked about, first in wonder and then with scattered tales of experience. All of the things that were undesirable around our family dining room table came alive at school and, in some cases, seemed more positive than my parents had ever let on.

Despite the talk, responsibility was what I increasingly felt as I traversed my teenage years. My mother spent a great deal of time reminding me that I was my brother's principal role model and the one he looked up to. Implied in those statements, always, was the command that I must live a life that Jon could safely emulate. I was not merely a role model for a younger brother; I was to be a role model for a younger brother with diabetes.

Some important research focuses on the relationship between siblings when one has a chronic disease such as diabetes. The last two decades have seen a substantial increase in studies focused on the effect that a chronic illness has on a healthy sibling. Not surprising, most of the studies conclude that the presence of a child with chronic disease has negative impacts on healthy siblings.[7] One study even concluded that when a child has a chronic disease or other serious illness, that child's healthy siblings often become the unhappiest and the most emotionally neglected members of the family.[8]

---

7   Donald Sharpe and Lucille Rossiter, "Siblings of Children with a Chronic Illness: A Meta-Analysis," *Journal of Pediatric Psychology* 27, no. 8 (December 2002): 699–710, http://jpepsy.oxfordjournals.org/content/27/8/699.full.pdf+html.
8   Samantha Suzanne Newcom, "Siblings of Chronically Ill Children" (master's report, University of Arizona, 2004), http://www.nursing.arizona.edu/Library/Newcom_SS.pdf.

Several studies have also identified an increased responsibility role as one of the paths that healthy siblings take when confronted with a chronically ill sibling.[9] This increased responsibility can deteriorate the sibling relationship and transform it into one resembling a parent–child relationship. This is what happened to Jon and me when I entered my high school years.

In my mind, the fact that my brother was diabetic made all the difference in the world when it came to my serving as his number one role model, as everyone around me assured me I was. If I was, in essence, to be Jon's hero, I had a responsibility to do so in a manner conducive to good diabetes management. I had to do things that were healthy and that Jon, as a person with diabetes, could safely do. I had to act as if I was a diabetic, and a perfectly managed one at that.

This was an impossible role for me to fill. I was not a diabetic. As a teenage boy, I had little desire to live a perfectly managed life. Even if I had wanted to, I did not know what that meant. What was acceptable behavior for a young diabetic? What were the healthy practices that my brother would need to follow when he found himself in the young adult situations that I was in? Which path would lead to health and safety? Which path could lead to more illness, maybe even death?

I knew that I did not have the answers to these questions. In some regard, as a rebellious teen, I did not care to learn the answers. Why should my actions be governed by the needs of my brother? I wanted to do what I wanted to do, whether my little brother could do so safely or not. It was my life after all.

---

9   Ibid.

The expectations for me were clear: excel in school and be a good role model for Jon. If I did not fulfill those roles, I would let my mother and father down. I would fail my family.

So, at the age of fourteen or so, I was faced with this major dilemma. To be a good son and a good brother I had to strive for perfection. In the opposite corner of my mind were of all my teenage hormones and my desire to be my own person. Between these two poles was the stark realization that I had few ideas about which elements of my life would be good or bad for Jon to emulate. Drug and alcohol use would of course be bad for me and probably worse for Jon. Everything else seemed vague. Would sex be bad for diabetics? Was an interest in girls good for my brother? There were a hundred similar questions.

In the end, I did the only thing I knew how to do - I compromised. I could not overcome the pressure to be my brother's hero, so I had to become that. But I convinced myself that I did not actually have to live that way. I would do what I wanted; I would hide all of me from Jon.

I decided that I would split into two. I would be the hero my little, diabetic brother thought I was and that my parents wanted me to be. At the same time, I would shield Jon from everything in my life that was not clearly good and acceptable within my family. If there was doubt, I would hide it. I would not stop doing anything because of Jon; I just would not let him into that side of my life.

I had little to hide in retrospect. My mother was quite successful in her efforts to raise polite, straight-laced, good kids. I did well academically and athletically throughout high school. I was a member of the National Honor Society and had little experience of the after-school detention hall. Drinking and drugs did not interest me. I may have had a couple of beers at the end of senior year — that was the extent of it.

I was a bit mischievous, but my mischief was almost always good, clean fun. I was not destructive and remained respectful of other people and their property. I did not throw eggs at Halloween or join the parties in the woods on Saturday nights.

Chasing girls became my biggest vice, if that can be considered a vice, during those years. Jon knew all three of my steady girlfriends during high school, but he didn't know details of our relationships. My relationships were presented as many parents presented theirs at the time: They existed and that was all Jon needed to know.

These efforts to keep Jon at a distance had a lasting impact. There was no sharing of secrets or stories between siblings. There were no locker room jokes. All intimacy between Jon and I was cast aside. I built a thick wall to hide something that had no need to be hidden. I just did not know that at the time.

I graduated from high school in the spring of 1990. I had been itching to graduate and move on to college since the middle of my sophomore year, so graduation was pure bliss. The wall between Jon and me was thick and strong with no gaps. When I packed for college later that same summer, the wall came with me.

After considerable internal debate, from the seven colleges where I was accepted, I chose to attend Union College, whose beautiful campus is enclosed within the city of Schenectady, New York. Schenectady was about three hours from my family, so my selection placed me out of immediate reach yet not too far from home.

Union College is a small liberal arts school that was founded in 1795. Class sizes ranged between four hundred and five hundred students when I attended the school, so there were never more than two thousand students on campus. Coming from a small town in upstate New York, Union's smallness was attractive.

Like most freshmen in college, it took me a while to adjust to the independence and freedom that I enjoyed when, for the first time in my life, I was not living under my parents' roof. Naturally, I went through a short period of homesickness during the first weeks of that first year. Most of my newfound friends and acquaintances did, though few of us would say so aloud.

I roomed that year with a high school classmate who had also decided that Union was the place to be for the next four years. We shared a small double room in South College, one of the older dormitories on campus and, at that time, all male. Though we were only acquaintances in high school, my roommate and I became fast friends that first year and soon found ourselves exploring one of Union's claims to fame — its Greek system.

Union College is known as the mother of fraternities. It earned this moniker by being the birthplace of the first three college fraternities, or secret societies, in the nation: Kappa Alpha, Sigma Phi Society, and Delta Phi. At Union, the term "frat" was never used.

I sampled most of the campus's dozen fraternities in the first weeks of my freshman year but found myself continually drawn to one — the Sigma Phi Society, founded in 1827. It was a good fit, and I fell in love with the society and its members. I pledged during the fall and winter of 1990 and was initiated as a member in the spring of 1991.

It was one of the best things I have done for myself. I blossomed at Union and at Sigma Phi. I became what at other institutions might be called a quintessential frat boy. I had a lot of fun.

Each of the fraternities had its own house, some a grand mansion and others the wing of a dorm. The houses were equipped with large bar-rooms in their basements or first floors. Beer flowed from keg systems and was free for all but the fraternity members, whose social dues provided the means for the ongoing party.

During my time at Union, students went "out," meaning they went to one or more fraternity barrooms, every night of the week except Sunday and Tuesday. We started at 11:00 p.m. and often made it to bed between 2:00 and 3:00 a.m. Unless someone had put an early morning class on his schedule, he did not rise until nine or ten on a weekday or noon on the weekend. On weekdays, there was no time for breakfast because we had to hustle to make our first class. Our first meal on those days was lunch. Lunch was followed by more classes, dinner, and either schoolwork or fun until 11:00 p.m., when the cycle started again.

It did not take a lot of thought to understand that skipping breakfast, sleeping until noon, and drinking plastic cup after plastic cup of beer was not exactly good for anyone, let alone my younger brother dealing with the additional challenges of diabetes. That understanding did not stop me from participating in the ritual. But because I was a role model for Jon, he could never know about this life that I, along with thousands of others across the country, led in college.

When I was home, the stories of college that I shared with Jon were, as they had been since high school: severely censored. My conversations about college with Jon involved the same tales about classes and innocuous activities that my parents received. There were no intimate secrets shared between brothers, no winks and nods.

Despite what I shared at home, I realized that if high school had opened the door into the world for me, college blew that door off its hinges. The country boy was exposed to a microcosm of the vast and varied society we live in. Even at the small elite college, I met peers from all walks of life and circumstances, far different from the homogenous little town in upstate New York where I had spent my first eighteen years.

At Union I found another freedom that I had never imagined. For the first time in eleven years, I could sleep through the night without any chance of being awoken by my brother's screams and the heavy running footsteps of my parents. Likewise, my days were free from anxiety about my brother's blood sugar level and all other aspects of diabetes.

College also freed me from diabetes management responsibilities. I was three hours away. There was nothing I could do to help my brother or my mother even if I wanted to. My role was reduced to hearing about a bad reaction or that everything was going fine during occasional telephone conversations with my mother. I was removed from the situation, and it felt wonderful.

My freedom from the fear and responsibility tied to my brother's diabetes disappeared at one point in my time at Union College. Union had been one of the early adopters of the philosophy that students should spend at least one term, or semester, studying abroad. I choose to spend the fall term of my junior year studying at the University of Bath in Bath, England. This was an incredible experience, and an opportunity that I am happy to have had.

When my parents blessed my plans to study in England, they also decided that my brother should travel over the Atlantic with me. The two of us were to travel through Europe two weeks before my classes in Bath began. Arrangements were made for Jon and me to fly with my Uncle Chris to Zurich, Switzerland, where Chris was studying at the Carl Jung Institute. With the help of my parents, my brother and I established our travel itinerary. Starting in Switzerland, we would make our way by train through Germany and the Netherlands and then cross the channel to spend our last few days together in London.

Jon and I were both ecstatic at the prospect of this European jaunt. At our respective ages of seventeen and twenty, we would be on our own in Europe. For me, though, the closer we came to our departure date, the more I realized that this trip was both exciting and terrifying. I would be alone with my diabetic brother, thousands of miles from home and parents.

It was to be just Jon and me on this huge trip. Our French was bad, our German and Dutch nonexistent. Other than Jon himself, when it came to his diabetes, I would be in charge. I would be the adult. If Jon had an insulin reaction or his blood sugar got too high, I would be the only one there to help him. These realizations were frightening.

Despite my fears, our trip was planned and was not going to be halted. On the appointed day, my family drove to Boston, our departure city. Jon, Chris, and I waved good-bye and boarded the plane that would carry us first to Brussels and then to Zurich. When the wheels retracted and the plane rose into the air, I was scared. I am sure my brother was too, and I can only begin to imagine how worried my mother was as she watched the plane leave the ground and turn toward the unknown.

Our trip through Switzerland, Germany, and the Netherlands was more spectacular than either Jon or I had imagined. The people we met were friendly, and the sites we saw amazing. Quicker than either of us had wanted, we found ourselves in London on the last day of the travels together. I put Jon on his plane home at Heathrow and took the train to Bath to begin my term abroad.

Jon and I made it through Europe without incident. There were no reactions and no dangerous high blood sugar events. We made sure we ate when Jon needed to, and he was careful to administer the proper doses of insulin commensurate with each day's planned activity level. Thousands of miles from home, we both had a great time and kept diabetes safely in control. I was pleased and proud of us both.

Despite our success with diabetes, the wall that I erected between Jon and me was not overcome during our travels abroad. I remember taking several private jaunts to avail myself of the more liberal European society while leaving him alone in our hotel room or at a hostel. Even thousands of miles from home, I was not going to allow Jon to see me in any way other than as an ideal role model. We conquered many fears and challenges that trip, but at the end I remained more of a parent than a brother.

At the end of my junior year at Union College, my brother graduated from the high school we had both attended. In the fall of my senior year, Jon began his four years of college at St. Lawrence University in Canton, New York. During the year that we were both college students, Jon visited me at Union a few times and I went to St. Lawrence to visit him.

Whether at Union or St. Lawrence, the wall was between us. When on my home turf, it was almost impossible for me to shield the life I lived from my brother. I had lived in the Sigma Phi house since sophomore year, staying there during the summers, as well as the academic year. When Jon visited during the school year, the house was in full swing and the barroom was packed.

Faced with the inability to shield Jon from these truths, I simply turned my back on my brother when he visited and stood aloof from him and the scene. Jon instead turned to my friends, and many soon became his friends as well. He had a good time during his visits to Union. It just was not with me.

The wall that I had spent most of my high school and college years constructing between my brother and my true self was a strong one. I hauled every brick to Boston University School of Law and kept it in place after Jon graduated from St. Lawrence and attended the New York College of Osteopathic Medicine. The wall's useful life was long expired, but neither of us knew how to take it down.

If the wall can be said to have had any effect, it most likely did so during my high school years, not while I was in college or law school. Jon is a smart guy. By the time I started college, he surely saw me for who I was. The wall I had hoped was opaque turned out to be quite transparent. But I am sure Jon never guessed why I had built the wall in the first place: to protect him and provide him with the perfect role model that I was pressured to be.

Chapter Fourteen

———✺———

PRESENT

On January 11, 2016, my brother marked the thirty-seventh anniversary of his diabetes diagnosis. He has successfully lived with the debilitating disease for more than three decades. Jon has never let diabetes stop him from doing what he wants to do.

Jon graduated from the New York College of Osteopathic Medicine in 2001 and completed his residency at Upstate Medical Center in Syracuse, New York. Much to the surprise of many of us, he chose to specialize in emergency medicine.

Following his residency in Syracuse, Jon returned home with his family and purchased our grandmother's house, just six miles down the road from where we grew up. Our grandmother had died in 2000, and my brother moved his family into the house with our great-aunt, Alfreda, who remained with them until she died at the age of ninety-two in January 2013.

Jon initially worked in the emergency room in the local hospital in

Plattsburgh and was one of the most popular doctors on staff. Feeling the urge to spread his wings, he seized the opportunity to purchase an urgent care practice in town when the previous owner reached retirement age, and Urgicare of the Northeast (now known as Beach Medical Services) was born. Though he had no prior business experience, my brother jumped into the practice and it has blossomed.

So far, Jon's urgent care practice has doubled in size at least twice and has added care centers devoted to allergies, weight loss, cardiology and of course, diabetes. The diabetes practice is one of the largest providers and trainers of insulin pumps in the Northeast, and my brother travels throughout the country to give training presentations.

Jon also serves as the presiding doctor for most of the local emergency medical services teams in his county and is often a first responder to emergency situations. He is trained in swift-water rescue, a skill that became personally important a few years ago when he rescued our father from a vehicle being washed away by floodwaters.

Deciding that running a successful medical practice was not enough, in 2011 my brother threw his hat in the local political ring. He successfully ran for a seat on the county legislature. Jon was sworn in on January 1, 2012, for a two-year term and won a second term when he ran unopposed in the fall of 2013. He has become a hardworking legislator and is popular among his constituents.

Most importantly, my brother is a proud father of two healthy and happy children. He is a devoted family man, who spends all of his spare time making sure that his family is safe and happy.

Jon's family became a bit larger three years ago, when it welcomed Banting, a chocolate Labrador retriever. Banting, named after one of the Canadian men who discovered insulin, is not a pet; he is a diabetes service dog. Trained to smell the difference between blood sugar levels since he was a puppy, Banting is on duty twenty-four hours a day, seven days a week, alerting my brother when his blood sugar swings low or high through a series of gestures. It is quite something to see.

~~~

Both of my parents are healthy and well. My mother is seventy-four years old and my father is sixty-nine. My mother still lives in the house that Jon and I grew up in. Jon's Cabin still stands in the back of the property. All of our children play in it when they visit.

My parents see Jon and his family quite a bit, though busy schedules make it less than one would think given their proximity. My mother still spends a good deal of her time worrying about my brother but is comforted with the presence of Banting who is quite adept at helping Jon manage his diabetes.

My relationship with my mother has never been better. Through time and the wisdom that seems to come from being a parent oneself, I have realized that Mom was placed in a very difficult situation and did her best to accommodate both of her sons. Because she is an amazing person with untold strength, her untiring efforts were immense. At the age of seventy-four, my mother is still going strong and still devoted to both Jon and me and our respective families. The distance that diabetes drove between my Mom and me has been vanquished, its poison removed. We are mother and son now, just as we were before that dreadful winter of 1980.

~~~

As I write this, I am forty-four years old and happy. I am married to Sarah, the love of my life, and have two beautiful children: Tristan, who is seventeen years old, and Colby, who is fourteen. These three people are the joy in my life.

After law school, I returned to Plattsburgh and hung up my shingle with a solo practitioner. I soon became the general counsel for Plattsburgh Airbase Redevelopment Corp. (PARC), a development company formed in 1995 to redevelop the former Plattsburgh Air Force Base, a vast, 3,500-acre facility.

Following three successful years at PARC, I relocated to New York's capital region in 2002 and joined the law firm of Whiteman Osterman & Hanna, where I remain today. I still have several clients in Plattsburgh, and I travel there often for work. When I can, I see Jon and my mom on those trips.

Tristan and Colby are my pride and joy. Like my brother and me, the boys are three years apart in age. Watching them grow up together, I often think of Jon and me. Tristan and Colby are best friends. They are constantly together. Though they both play and bicker like all brothers, they sure seem to fight a whole lot less than Jon and I did.

My boys are healthy, and for that I am eternally thankful. Their relationship prospers and grows without the dark cloud of diabetes or another chronic condition. Tristan has a normal sense of responsibility toward his younger brother, and without effort or pressure, he is an excellent role model for Colby. My sons are not burdened with the responsibility, jealousy, resentment, and fear that marked my relationship with my brother. There is no debilitating wall between them.

My sons are simply brothers. Seeing them together brings home how diabetes destroyed my sibling relationship with Jon. In retrospect, the decision to block Jon from the realities of my life was one of the worst I have made. Once I started building the wall between us, it never stopped, and it has stood between the two of us for nearly thirty years. It is only recently that I have begun to tear it down.

Tearing down the wall is not an easy task. It is not as simple as declaring "The wall is gone" and then standing back and watching it disappear. Instead, I am finding that nearly thirty years of a learned and practiced behavior is a lot to overcome.

Even as two adults, the idea of getting together with my brother always sounded good but usually turned out poorly. I was excited to see Jon on the drive to his house. I was excited until I walked through his door. Then the wall came back as if on autopilot. My smile was dismissed, and I became cold to Jon and his family. I could not let them in, and I dared not venture much beyond the surface of their lives. Each time I saw Jon, no matter where or what the circumstances, this pattern prevailed. Each visit ended disappointingly for both of us.

The tragedy of our story is that despite my refusal to let Jon into my life, I love my brother very much. Diabetes and I, not a lack of love, were the co-creators of the separation between Jon and me. Diabetes has no care whether the wall between us remains or crumbles. I do. And no one else can or will tear that wall down for me. The pages you have just read are part of my attempt to do just that.

I hope that Jon will realize someday why I did what I did. I was always a responsible person, but diabetes pressured me to be more responsible at a young age than anyone should be. I hope my brother will someday know that I tried to be responsible and to protect him from everything that would cause him harm. I want him to understand that I truly believed I was going where he should not.

Most of all, I hope that, when I do manage to tear away the last brick between us, my brother is standing there and that we are simply brothers again. The two men who face each other will not be boys of twelve and nine, but perhaps I will still slip him a note that says, "I am sorry, let's play." I believe that he will answer "okay."

PART THREE
OBSERVATIONS
AND WORDS OF ADVICE

Chapter Fifteen

———∞———

TELLING OUR STORY

Because you are reading this book, you may have some connection to diabetes or another dreadful chronic illness that strikes young people. Perhaps you are a mother or father of a chronically ill child. Perhaps you are that chronically ill child. Or maybe you are like me, the healthy sibling of a chronically ill brother or sister.

Regardless of your connection to the topic, I hope that this book has brought into focus the disruption that chronic diseases, such as diabetes, cause within families — particularly their impacts on healthy siblings. Managing a chronic disease within the family structure is a challenge. The type of disease matters little. A young child struck with disease changes each and every facet of family life. Families have no choice: With the diagnosis, the disease forces itself into the family. It is unwelcome, and it never leaves.

For a long time, the healthy siblings within families forced to face the challenges of a chronically ill child have been largely ignored. As one of these shadow children, I am intimately familiar with this near neglect by all who are concerned with chronic illness and children.

The writing of this book is the culmination of many hours of introspection. When I began, I was not sure what I would say or why I felt the need to put my thoughts in writing. I just knew that I wanted to. I now know that writing this book was a necessary step toward tearing down the wall between my brother Jon and me and repairing the relationship between us.

I am also aware that the story of my family's struggle with the unwelcome specter called diabetes is not unique. Details and personalities differ, but the hundreds of thousands of families that deal with a chronically ill child have similar stories. Be it diabetes, cancer, or some other loathsome disease, the chronically ill child changes families forever. In sharing the story of my family, I hope to offer families now struggling with illness, and those that will do so in the future, a bit of assurance that they are not alone — and perhaps a bit of wisdom and the courage to change and share their own story.

Chapter Sixteen

———— ✎ ————

WHAT I HAVE LEARNED

This year marked the thirty-seventh anniversary of my brother's diagnosis. I am always mindful to give possession of that diagnosis to my brother. It is Jon who bears the physical scars and fights the ongoing battle with diabetes. It is as if the two, my brother and the disease, are locked in an unending wrestling match. Sometimes my brother has the advantage; often diabetes does. Barring a miraculous cure, the match will continue until my brother's death. I hope that in the end, my brother dies naturally of old age and does not give that villainous disease the pleasure of winning the match.

Though the anniversary of the diagnosis is most directly felt by Jon, it does not go unnoticed by the rest of our family or closest friends. Jon has not been alone in this three-decades-long struggle with diabetes. My parents and I have been there too, and we have been more than mere spectators. We all quietly mark the diagnosis anniversary, for it was a turning point for all of us.

Every cloud has a silver lining. That is what they say. So what is the silver lining within the dark diabetes cloud that has hung over my family for years? I cannot answer that question for my parents or my brother. For me, the answer is simply that there is not a silver lining. The disease, like all chronic illnesses, is a terrible one. It has hurt my brother daily since he was four years old. It has hurt my mother and father. It has hurt me. At best, it is managed. It is never conquered.

If there is no silver lining, than the next question has to be: Has diabetes taught me anything? To this question, I can respond with a resounding yes. Watching my brother suffer and manage diabetes, and being a part of his management team for many years, taught me a great deal. Some of this "knowledge" imparted by chronic disease is general, such as increased senses of empathy and responsibility. Other things I have learned along this journey are specific to the effects of chronic disease on families.

I lack formal training in sociology, psychology, and family dynamics. I am not a doctor, nor do I play one on TV. I am an attorney and a writer. What I know about diabetes and its impact on families is through firsthand experience. But like street smarts, I believe that my experiences and knowledge have value, so I offer my observations in the pages that follow.

The disease is a member of the family, forever.

After one member of a family is diagnosed with a chronic disease, the entire family returns to a home that is familiar but forever changed. There is a new member of the family on that day. The disease is not a guest. It will not leave. It will be present at every meal and every event. The disease tags along on trips to the grocery store and on family vacations. It refuses to be left behind.

As a member of the family, the chronic disease does not belong to just its bodily host; it belongs to every member of the family. The disease is an equal-opportunity player when it comes to impacts. Its direct target is the subject of the diagnosis, but the disease digs its razor-sharp claws into each member of the family. It rapidly changes the lives of all.

By definition, the target of a chronic disease will not know a life without its presence. Yet the disease will remain with the parents of a chronically ill child for the rest of their lives too. They will not have a home in which the disease is absent. When a chronically ill child like my brother leaves home, attends college, and lives a separate adult life, part of the disease remains at home with his mother and father. Even a healthy sibling like me does not leave the chronic disease behind as he grows up and leaves home. The disease travels with the healthy sibling too. It invades his adult life and sits alongside him when he settles into his own home.

Another example of these superpowers that the disease as family member has is its ability to continually extend its reach, affecting the loved ones of each family member. As the chronic disease travels with each family member, it affects the lives of their respective loved ones and intimates.

Boyfriends and girlfriends of a young person with a chronic disease will be affected, and any future spouse will be forced to embrace the disease and adopt the lifestyle it demands. This seems obvious. Less obvious is that the loved ones and intimates of a healthy sibling are also subject to the talons of the chronic disease.

Becoming close to the healthy sibling means learning about the chronic disease that inflicts the family member. Not only are the intimates, loved ones, spouses, and children of the healthy sibling affected by knowledge of the disease, they are also affected by the scars that the disease has left on the healthy sibling. After all, the chronic disease has played a major role in the formation of the healthy sibling's psyche. The disease is part of the healthy sibling and so directly effects, and in many cases interferes with, each relationship the healthy sibling has with others.

Parents do the best they can in a horrible situation.

Let's face it; parenting is the toughest job you'll ever have. I have two boys, seventeen and fourteen, and I have my hands full. Being a dad is the greatest thing I have ever experienced. It is also the hardest and most demanding. I say that even as the father of two boys who are well-behaved, young gentlemen and, above all, healthy.

The addition of a chronic illness into the long list of demands and responsibilities placed on modern-day parents must be nearly un-bearable. Even though I grew up with parents who faced this extreme challenge daily, I still find it hard to fathom. Yet as parents, we all do what we have to do for our children. We don't give up. We don't walk away when the challenges become greater. We just march on, doing our best.

Looking back at my experience as a healthy sibling to a chronically ill child, it would be all too easy for me to cast stones at my parents for the wrongs, both real and perceived, that I felt throughout those years. As an adult and parent, though, I know that doing so would be an expression of misguided anger. It would also be terribly unfair to two parents who did the best they could in terrible circumstances.

Mothers and fathers are humans, with limitations and imperfections. As children, we sometimes forget this. A mother has only so much time and so much energy to devote to her children. No matter how amazing a person is, the resources of an individual are limited. If a mother has a young child whose chronic illness demands most of her time and attention, the other children in the family will have less of her time and attention. Fathers are no different. It is simple math.

The introduction of a chronic childhood disease into a family represents a significant challenge to parents. The family structure changes. Parenting styles change to meet the new demands. The apple cart will be upset; there is no way around it. The old family routines will be thrown out the door. With these changes, healthy siblings will suffer. Mother and father will devote more time and attention to the sick child. It is natural and to be expected.

For healthy siblings reading this book, I ask you to step back from your situation and appreciate these words. If you are older, and perhaps a parent yourself, understanding them is likely to come more easily to you. If you are still young, try to put yourself in the shoes of your parents. Your parents love you. They are doing their best. It's just that their best is not good enough. It can't be. They are in an impossible situation: They want to devote time and attention to you as they once did, but the health and survival of their sick child won't allow them to do that.

Mothers and fathers handle chronic illness differently.

Our society pushes a unisex message about all things in life. Today, the ideal woman is often the same as the ideal man. Fathers do tasks once considered only fit for mothers, and vice versa. Much has changed from my childhood of three decades ago. As a father, I do things around the house and with my children that my own father would not have dreamed of doing.

Our roles as mothers and fathers have intertwined, and overall this is a good thing. In the case of a chronic disease like diabetes, this means that today's fathers are more likely to be available and willing to pick up the slack left from the mother's required attention to her child's diabetes management. I can only imagine how much of a positive effect this has in their households.

Yet there are still many differences between men and women, mothers and fathers. Mothers and fathers react differently to the challenges presented by a chronically ill child. They also react differently to the healthy siblings. This can be a positive thing too.

My relationship with my father grew following Jon's diagnosis. My mother had to devote herself to Jon's care. My father was helpful but was the second team, so to speak. With my mother's attention turned almost completely to my brother, I turned to my father.

However, unless there is good communication within the family, family members tend to split into factions. The son who receives all of his attention from the father naturally aligns with the father and begins to resent the mother. This can lead to disaster, to say the least.

Families need to recognize the difference between mothers and fathers and their respective roles in the family with respect to the sick and healthy children alike. Mothers and fathers who work as a team, who communicate well with each other and their children, are likely to find dealing with the challenges of chronic illnesses more manageable. In these families, the healthy siblings stand a better chance of avoiding the emotional neglect that so often comes with the territory.

Siblings are severely affected but often forgotten.

The introduction of a chronic disease into the family unit wreaks havoc within the family structure and does not spare the healthy sibling. I hope that the stories contained within these pages, my stories, illustrate the severe impact that chronic illness had on me even though I was a healthy child.

The chronic disease attacks healthy siblings with unending feelings guilt in the form of self-blame and survivor's guilt. Diabetes and other chronic diseases also plant seeds of jealousy and resentment and create situations that nourish those seeds. At the same time, they force the healthy sibling to become more responsible at a very early age.

Chronic diseases such as diabetes also breed fear within healthy siblings. I became deeply afraid that I was on the verge of losing my brother at an early age. I lived with the fear that he might die. I dreaded my brother's insulin reactions and became afraid to be alone with him.

Guilt, resentment, and fear were poisons that diabetes injected into me. The poisonous thoughts became part of my life and lasted well beyond my childhood and teenage years. Through this poisoning, the "healthy sibling" label became a misnomer. Physically, I was fine, but inside I became very unhealthy.

In most cases, the severe impacts of chronic disease on healthy children go unnoticed. With the bulk of their attention and caregiving necessarily devoted to the inflicted child, parents often fail to recognize the effects that the disease has on their healthy children. The outward manifestations of these impacts are easily cast aside through labels such as "annoying" or mistakenly chalked up to "childlike behavior" that will be outgrown.

Healthy siblings are left to stew in the toxic thoughts and feelings that the disease has implanted within their psyche. The poisons become embedded in the personality, self-esteem, and inner foundation that form and grow during the early years of life. Healthy children will not outgrow these impacts. Instead, they taint all of our social and intimate relationships throughout life.

Chronic disease alters the sibling relationship.

When my brother was diagnosed with diabetes in 1980, he ceased being simply my brother. On that day, Jon became my brother who had diabetes. Our relationship was significantly altered from that day forward. I no longer thought of just Jon, but instead thought of Jon and diabetes.

As young children, all of our routines changed. This included how we played and interacted with each other. We could no longer play outside all day without being aware of mealtimes and snack times. If we went to The Rock or to Jon's Cabin, we both needed to have honey packets in our pockets in case Jon's blood sugar dropped.

The responsibility I felt, as the healthy child, stunted our relationship as brothers. I could no longer be just a brother; I had to adopt many of the responsible stances that come with parenthood. This eventually led me to build a wall to protect Jon from everything I thought might cause him harm. He was no longer my best friend and confidant, and I was no longer his. I was his third parent, watching over him and protecting him but not sharing the intimacies of life with him.

While different children adopt various defenses and coping mechanisms as healthy siblings, in all cases their relationship with their sick brother or sister permanently changes. This is an unavoidable consequence of chronic disease.

Disease alters every other family relationship.

Diabetes drove a wedge between my mother and me. My mother was my brother's primary caregiver. She had to take care of her sick child above all else. Between a diabetic son and a healthy son, the needs of the diabetic son had to come first. My mother was aware of this; she felt guilty then, and she feels that guilt to this day. What she most likely was not aware of was the extent of the toxic impact that diabetes was having on me.

Fortunately, my grandmother, and great-aunt were there for me day after day. Through these two adults, I recaptured some of what I had lost with my mother and brother. It is hard for me to imagine my life being as good as it was without that support system. I am sure that healthy siblings who are not as fortunate have a tougher time.

Diabetes also changed the relationships Jon had with other members of our family. As his primary caregiver, my mother became extremely close to Jon, forming a tight bond that exists to this day. At the same time, while I was always available to join my father at work or on some adventure, Jon was not.

Sadly, members of our family outside of our household allowed their ignorance and fear of diabetes to effectively end their relationship with my brother. I know words such as "I don't have time for your problems" were cast more than once in my brother's direction. While it was easy to have me over for a day or night, people were not so ready to take in both Jon and diabetes.

Chronic disease also altered the relationship between my parents. My parents' relationship is far beyond the scope of my experience and reflection, but I am confident that they both have much to share about the impacts that diabetes had on them as individuals and as a couple.

Chapter Seventeen

WORDS FOR PARENTS

As I have made clear, I am not a psychologist or physician. I have no formal training on the human mind or family relationships. What I do have is thirty-seven years of experience as the sibling of a diabetic. I also have thirty-seven years of experience living within a family forced to accept chronic disease as family member and part of daily life. It is my experience, rather than training, that I draw upon in offering the following words of advice and caution.

Do not forget your healthy children and their needs.

There is no question about it: Being a parent of a child with a chronic disease is incredibly difficult. If the chronic disease requires daily monitoring and management, as so many do, your task is even harder. Your chronically ill child's needs are exponentially increased, requiring you to devote a tremendous amount of resources and energy toward that child. Many parents also quickly find all of their worries and concerns exponentially increased for the sick child.

Parental focus on the chronically ill child is natural and, indeed, necessary. What I beseech you to do is to recognize the inevitable imbalance of attention that occurs between sick and healthy children. Recognize that imbalance, and communicate your recognition with your healthy children. Let them know that you realize you are spending more time with the sick child and are more attentive to their needs, and let them know why this is necessary.

This simple act of communication will accomplish a couple of important things. First, communicating with your healthy children tells them that you have not forgotten them. As a parent, it may seem silly to think that this needs to be reinforced for a child, but it does. Chronic illness is so demanding that it is easy for healthy children to feel forgotten and left in the shadows.

By communicating with the healthy children about the attention imbalance, its necessity, and its unfairness, you tell those children that they matter. Even if healthy children are very young and may not understand completely, such communication and such recognition of the unfairness of the situation will help them realize that they are not the reason for the attention imbalance.

Honest communication regarding your limited resources and the demands of the chronic disease will also open up a dialogue between you and your healthy children about what is happening and how they are feeling. Again, the communication reinforces that they are not forgotten. Such discussions may also lead to ways to meet some, if not all, of the needs that a healthy child feels are being neglected. Through these conversations, you will discover how the healthy child perceives the situation and perhaps find ways to make your child feel more included.

Accept that there are now limits to what you can give a healthy child.

You should not try to be superhuman and act as if you are capable of retaining the balance of attention and care that was present within the family before the diagnosis of chronic illness. We all want to be everything to our children, but even in healthy families this is a dream. Parents who have a chronically ill child cannot possibly care for that child without taking time and attention away from their healthy children.

Accepting these limits is often easier said than done, especially for mothers. What mother wants to admit that she cannot care for all of her children at the same level? Mothers want to believe that they can do anything it takes for their children. In a family with a chronically ill child, this belief and related stubbornness are likely to be counterproductive. Equality is impossible. You are not less of a mother if you have to give up time with your healthy child because your sick child needs you. You are simply a normal human with limited resources.

Allowing yourself to be a human parent rather than pretending you are superhuman will open up opportunities for your healthy children. Just realizing you are not capable of achieving a balance of attention will help reveal the impacts of disease on these children. It may also help you avoid the otherwise inevitable guilt. Finally, such recognition will help you reach out to other family members and adults who can jump in occasionally and provide support for the healthy children.

Do not think that the family is unaltered or can weather the storm simply by continuing to do what it has always done.

As a parent, you must recognize early on that your family has been changed forever. Just as your ill child and that child's needs were forever changed on the day of diagnosis, so was your family. The old ways will not work with the demands of disease.

This realization may take some time. Faced with the unknowns of a chronic disease, we are likely to seek the familiar in our family structure and hold on tightly. This is only natural. Change is hard. Change is scary.

Unfortunately, the new member of your family, the chronic disease, has no patience. The disease demands immediate changes with respect to the routines of the sick child. These changes will affect the routines of every other family member as well. Pretending that the family structure can remain the same after diagnosis is counterproductive.

As difficult as it is, you must embrace the adjustments that the disease demands. Communication remains key. The reconfiguration of family structure and routine will be daunting to the healthy children, as well as to the ill one. Don't let that reconfiguration occur without a serious dose of communication. Let the healthy children know why things have to change. Help them find ways to adopt the changes and have their own needs met within the new family structure.

Chapter Eighteen

WORDS FOR HEALTHY SIBLINGS

You are not alone; there are thousands of us.

When my brother began spending his summers at the Camp Joslin, a diabetic camp in Massachusetts, one of camp's selling points was that young diabetic boys often felt alone, as if they were the only ones waking up each morning with diabetes. One of its goals was to reassure young boys with diabetes that there were many boys just like them.

While there is no summer camp dedicated to us, the healthy siblings of children with chronic illnesses, it is equally important that we understand we too are not alone. Just as there are thousands of children who face chronic illnesses daily, there are thousands of healthy siblings forced to endure the impacts of chronic illnesses.

I am not aware of formal support groups for the siblings of children with diabetes and other chronic illnesses. Perhaps it is time for such groups to be formed alongside the many support groups that exist to address each of the chronic diseases and their direct victims. In the meantime, we as healthy siblings should not feel alone. We are not the first ones to feel resentment or fear because of disease. We are not the only ones who feel overburdened with responsibilities that we are too young to bear, let alone understand.

We have all had to deal with these poisons of disease while being labeled the "lucky ones." We have been stabbed with pangs of guilt over circumstances beyond our control. There is no need to feel alone.

Work to understand your parents are only human and have limited resources.

Just as it is critical for parents of children with chronic illnesses to be honest with themselves and recognize that they are not superhumans, that understanding is important for us as healthy siblings. A seven-year-old boy is unlikely to grasp this concept, but teenagers can.

I can vouch for this being difficult at times. Even looking back from adulthood, it is sometimes hard to remember that your parents did the best they could in splitting themselves between your needs and the needs of your sick sibling. The fog of jealousy, resentment, and fear is often thick and difficult to pierce.

Despite the difficulties, the effort to achieve this understanding and remember it during difficult times is well worth it. Realizing and accepting this truth can ease the pain and frustration and even act as a bit of antivenom to the toxins of the disease that constantly invade our psyche.

Seek help from other family members, friends, and mentors to get in a healthy manner what your parents cannot give you.

Even understanding that your parents are doing the best they can, as a healthy sibling you will feel an absence. It may be a yearning for how things were in your family before your brother's or sister's diagnosis. It may be the absence of attention from one or both of your parents. It may be the absence of feeling safe and living without fear and dread. In many cases, it will be a combination of all of these things. Regardless, you will feel a hole within you and identify needs that are not being fully met.

Faced with this hole, you will naturally try to fill it. No one likes to walk around feeling incomplete. Everyone seeks to fulfill their needs when they are not met by their family structure. There are both unhealthy and healthy ways to fill these needs.

I sought to replace the attention I missed from my mother with attention from girlfriends. Beginning in my teenage years and continuing into young adulthood, I became quickly attached to the women who showed interest in me and entered into exclusive relationships with them. I was so happy to find what I erroneously believed to be a substitute that I would make heavy emotional investments in these unwitting companions. When these relationships ended, as they always did until my marriage, I would be crushed. The hole not only reappeared; it became larger. I felt rejected again and again, even when I was the party doing the breaking up, leading to feelings of unworthiness.

My nonromantic relationships were the healthy mechanism that I used to fill the hole created by diabetes. I was fortunate enough to have my grandmother and great-aunt close by. These two women stepped in as surrogate parents time after time. They were sources of company and emotional support when my mother was occupied with caring for my brother. My bonds with each of them became exceptionally strong and remained that way until their respective deaths.

I also found support from several other adults throughout my early years. Some of these mentors were teachers or coaches; others were family friends. Each helped and supported me in different ways, and each was a critical ally in my own fight against the poisons of chronic disease.

Whether it is family members outside of your immediate family or unrelated adult mentors, the importance of finding and surrounding yourself with this extraneous support group cannot be overstated. There is no need for formal explanations of your needs. You probably could not articulate them if you tried. The person you are looking for does not need explanations. The supporting relationship will develop naturally over time and will become one that you cherish.

Remember that you are a sibling, not a parent.

There is nothing wrong with being a responsible child, teenager, and young adult — we need more of those. There is also nothing wrong with pitching in to care for your brother or sister with a chronic disease. As a family member, it is to be expected. What must be avoided, though, is taking on more responsibility than can rightfully be expected of a healthy sibling.

As healthy siblings, we must take care to remain siblings and avoid becoming a third parent to an ill brother or sister. This is something that I, and many other healthy siblings, have failed to do. Yet you have the right to remain a child and be a brother or sister.

In part, this requires good communication. Tell your parents when you feel overwhelmed with responsibility toward your sibling. Let them know that you are happy to help out but that you cannot be a third adult within the family structure.

Your brother or sister needs a sibling and all of the intimate sharing that the sibling relationship brings with it. Finding the balance between helpful family member and third parent can be challenging, but in the long run you and your sibling will be happier if you can strike that balance.

Push back on guilt; this is not your fault.

My guilt began the day my brother was diagnosed. At seven years old, I was positive that my brother had diabetes because I picked on him too much. I wasn't quiet about it either. I told my father and my grandmother the same day. Jon was sick, and it was my fault.

As I grew up, my conviction that I was the cause of Jon's disease dissipated, but my feelings transformed from causal guilt to survivor's guilt. I felt guilty that I got out of bed each morning without having to look forward to at least two daily insulin injections. I felt guilty that there were no limits on my diet. I even felt guilty when people remarked how tall I was, knowing that my brother's growth had been stunted by not one but two autoimmune diseases.

All of these guilty feelings were without foundation. No action or inaction gave rise to the circumstances that my family found itself in. The situation was blameless. I knew that and still felt guilty.

That guilt seems to be universal among healthy siblings, as well as many other family members. I hope that you learn from my experience and do everything you can to stop feeling guilty. Your guilt is part of the chronic disease's package of poisons. They are destructive and will adversely affect all areas of your life.

When I finally confronted my guilt over Jon's diabetes, the act of communicating these feelings to others became my most successful defense against them. By talking with others whose opinions I respected and sharing my long-standing guilt with them, I started to free myself from these poisonous thoughts. In airing my feelings, I heard from others how misplaced those feelings were. Their support helped bring clarity to the blamelessness of chronic disease.

We are all different, and what works for me may not rid you of the poison of guilt. Communicating your feelings is always a good start though. Like the chronic disease itself, there is no absolute cure for its ancillary poisons. There are still moments when I feel elements of guilt creeping back in. The important thing is to learn to fight those erroneous feelings and rid yourself of as much of their presence as possible. Start early on this and work on it. Don't wait as I did. Start now.

Jealousy and resentment are natural and unavoidable; it's your job to make sure they do not overwhelm you.

My guess is that every healthy sibling carries the weight of jealousy of and resentment toward a brother or sister who has a chronic disease. I feel confident in making this guess because it is an educated one. My life experience and review of the available literature and studies regarding siblings and chronic diseases support this assertion.

It is natural — and unavoidable — for you as a healthy sibling to feel jealous or resentful of your sick brother or sister. These two negative emotions are, again, part of the poisonous package that chronic disease brings. The disease physically attacks your sibling and psychologically attacks you and other healthy family members.

To fight these poisons, you must first admit to your feelings toward your chronically ill sibling and recognize that they are natural. You are not some kind of monster because you become jealous when your sick sister receives more attention then you at home or your ill brother receives a seemingly unending stream of get-well cards and gifts long after leaving the hospital. You are not a horrible person because you resent certain privileges given only to your sick sibling. You are a normal human faced with the challenges of chronic disease.

Once you recognize your jealousy and resentment, you need to find ways to ensure that these feelings do not overwhelm you. In short, just as your sibling needs to manage the physical impacts of the disease, you need to manage the psychological impacts it is having on you.

Again, I don't have all of the answers on how to manage these feelings. For me, the first step is always communication. Find someone to talk to about your jealousy and resentment. Make sure that person is a good listener. If you express these feelings to someone and they act surprised or react with hostility toward you, the "lucky" one, then quickly move on and find someone else to talk to. The right listener will hear your concerns and empathize without judgment.

Always remember that jealousy and resentment are poisons fed to us by chronic diseases such as diabetes. It is natural to feel those emotions, but you don't get a free pass. Take control of your negative thoughts and manage them so that they do not become overwhelming forces within your life.

Remember that you have a right to live your life.

It can be easy to become so involved in the management and care that surrounds the sick sibling that your own life is forced into second place. Chronic illness can be a whirlwind, sucking the lives of all family members toward its center. Parents are unavoidably sucked into this vacuum. Healthy siblings can, and should, avoid this fate.

To remain a healthy sibling, you must have your own life. This means that you must have an independent life beyond the chronic disease that has inflicted your sister or brother and has so severely affected your family.

You are not a parent. You are a sibling. You have responsibilities toward your sick brother or sister, your parents, and your family unit. Those responsibilities have limits, though, and as I learned, they cannot be allowed to rise to the parental level.

By all means, be responsible and helpful. Just make sure that your role ends at the sibling limit and does not cross into the parental level. You will know when you get close to the limit. You will feel inside that something is not right.

Keeping within the sibling limits will allow you to live your own life. Have compassion and empathy, but do not allow yourself to be hand-cuffed to your sibling's fate. Live the life you want to live. Be you.

Remember that you are loved and make sure you love yourself.

The final advice that I offer to healthy siblings is to remember that you are loved and to love yourself. Heeding all of the preceding advice will make loving yourself and realizing you are loved easier. If you can defend against the poisons that diseases such as diabetes seek to im-plant within you, you will find it easier to love yourself. If you see your parents as the fallible humans they are, it will be easier to look past the attention imbalance and see that your parents love you very much.

In contrast, allowing the poisons of chronic disease to invade your life and permeate your mind will make recognizing external sources of love and self-love difficult. Poisons such as jealousy, resentment, and fear are not conducive to loving oneself. Those negative feelings will taint your vision of yourself, family, and other aspects of your life if you allow them to do so. Being overwhelmed with extra sibling responsibility and guilt will stunt your growth as an independent and whole person.

Your parents love you. They love you as much today as they did when you were born. Your parents would do anything they could to restore the attention balance that is disrupted by chronic disease. Unfortunately, the disease is too demanding, and your parents do not have a lot of options. You must see this. You must work to understand and feel their love. It is there.

As a healthy sibling, you must also learn or relearn self-love. Do not let the poisons of chronic disease overwhelm you and turn self-love into indifference or, worse, self-loathing. Face and name each of the poisons: guilt, fear, jealousy, resentment, excessive responsibility, and so on. Recognizing these invaders and talking with others about each of them will help you defend against their poison and develop your self-love.

You are not alone. You are loved. You are worthy.

Step out of the shadows.

EPILOGUE

The stories recounted here of my childhood as a healthy sibling to my diabetic brother began some thirty years ago in the late 1970s and 1980s. While diabetes remains as incurable today as it was then, there have been significant technological breakthroughs in the day-to-day management of the disease.

When my brother was diagnosed with diabetes, insulin was administered solely through injections. Luckily for my brother, these injections were administered through a sharp, disposable syringe with a thin plastic tube. Diagnosis a decade before would have meant a thicker, glass syringe that had to be boiled before each shot and resulted in a larger impact site.

Today my brother, along with thousands of other people with diabetes, has abandoned daily syringes. Instead, these diabetics receive a continuous subcutaneous insulin infusion through the use of an insulin pump. The pump uses sensors to regulate and administer insulin directly into the bloodstream. This device, no larger than a smartphone, saves diabetics from thousands of needle pricks over a lifetime.

The insulin that is pumped into my brother's body has also changed through the years. In the beginning, his treatment involved the administration of two types of insulin, regular insulin and neutral protamine of Hagedorn (NPH) insulin. NPH insulin was longer acting than regular insulin. Both types were derived from either cows or pigs. In the 1980s, breakthroughs in recombinant DNA technology resulted in the production of human insulin. Today's insulin is purer and more powerful than ever. It also comes in several longer- and rapid-acting forms.

Monitoring blood glucose levels in the early 1980s meant peeing into a small plastic container and putting a test strip in the urine for a minute. This monitoring was not incredibly accurate, giving only a range of glucose levels in the urine (not the blood). To obtain an accurate blood sugar reading, diabetics were required to visit the hospital for substantial blood work.

Sometime in the middle of the 1980s, my parents purchased an expensive blood monitor. Instead of peeing on a stick, this new monitor allowed my brother to directly test the amount of glucose in his blood. By sticking the tips of his fingers with a lancet and placing dabs of blood on a special test stick, which was then fed into the monitor, my brother could see a digital readout of his current blood sugar level.

Blood glucose monitors are now commonplace, are increasingly accurate, and require an ever-smaller blood sample. Many of these machines do not even require specialized test strips and are as small as pens, rather than the desk calculator–size devices my brother first used. The evolution of these machines has resulted in better diabetes management and fewer trips to the hospital blood lab.

Several continuous glucose monitoring (CGM) systems are also available on today's market. Similar to insulin pumps, these CGM systems are subcutaneous and do not require the continual puncturing of the skin. CGM systems allow diabetics to monitor their glucose levels continuously throughout the day and night.

Even the way diabetics eat has changed since my brother's diagnosis. Thirty years ago, diabetics used American Diabetes Association food exchange books with food lists and carbohydrate values. Food scales were used to learn to measure proper amounts of each of the allowable food groups. Meals were prescribed, and the insulin dose was fixed based on those meals. This meant that once the insulin was given, my brother had to eat the meal that was planned, even if he was not hungry or did not like the food. Today, the diet of the person with diabetes is less prescribed. Insulin can now be taken before or after meals, or continuously using an insulin pump, and are regulated based on what is actually eaten.

All of these changes in technology, together with our increased understanding of diabetes and its effects on the human body, have resulted in the ability to more carefully monitor and manage diabetes daily. While some of the technological changes have only made diabetes management different, many have made it easier.

These advances mean that the impact of diabetes on the family has also changed. A family with a child diagnosed with diabetes today has many more treatment options compared with those available to my family.

Despite these advances, diabetes remains a disease that requires constant vigilance. Modern medical literature suggests that with most conditions, patients are considered to be compliant with prescribed treatment if they take their medication at least 80 percent of the time.[10] Diabetes demands 100 percent compliance. Anything less leads to severe complications and hospital stays.

---

10 Marie T. Brown and Jennifer K. Bussell, "Medication Adherence: WHO Cares?" *Mayo Clinic Proceedings*, 86, no. 4 (April 2001): 304–14, http://www.ncbi.nlm. nih.gov/pmc/articles/PMC3068890.

I believe it is too early to tell whether these technological advances have lessened the impact of diabetes on healthy siblings. The poisons of excessive responsibility, guilt, fear, jealousy, and resentment are still present. As with the underlying disease, improvements in technology and treatment do not erase the need for awareness and management of these poisons.

Only the cure of chronic diseases such as diabetes will eliminate their poisonous effect on both ill and healthy siblings. Until such cures are realized, we must all march on with awareness and diligence.